Mr. Haute Coiffure

Amazon Edition
ISBN: 978-1533515131

design: Eric Doctor

MR. HAUTE COIFFURE

BY JEHR SCHIAVO
WRITING AS GERARD SAINT D'ANGELO

✛

INTRODUCTION

Lazy publishers and their nonsense directives expect
us budding writers to deliver copy for inside jacket
alongside back cover; this hatching alone can make or
break a book's success. A perfectly sublime author's
work might easily slip away, going south if three points
of interest don't leave readers curious enough to desire
more; those embodied parameters: about said author,
book's elevator synopsis, and who's endorsing it.

The Ten Commandments seem reasonable, listing certain
rules to abide by; yet if I were some reformed philanderer,
thief, or murderer-turned-writer, most in drove-loads could
hardly wait before peering into my manuscript — but I'm not.

Charlton Heston didn't hike down Cecil B. DeMille's
mountain holding an extra large Wheaties-size stone
tablet with inscribed divine warning against illegal drugs;
nonetheless, lucky me, I eventually stopped using — they
simply took up too much time. There, ya happy now? I
know, almost straight away the devil inside asked yourself,
"How far did he go?"

Of course, human nature is complicated, though mine a career styling hair, remaining up close and ultra personal with clients did narrow the playing field. By many respects Marianne Faithfull should've stayed closer to Brian Jones; confiding in me, she softly quivered, "perhaps that entire unfortunate ordeal, his untimely drowning, may have not occurred," still dabbing her tears after thirty-three years, while on tour cutting Marianne's hair within an old-world George V, Paris Empire Suite.

Which tale, though, is more believable?

Vietnam Purple Heart recipient Teddy Toth, later becoming New York City Hells Angels Chapter's elder statesman, arriving for his San Francisco Jehrcut, requesting a look less obtrusive for upcoming obligatory air travel plans — specifically toying with FBI and ATF nosing around. Afterward, Teddy and I reminisced about delta bluesman John Campbell, whom we both considered a brother, over my fresh brew of Peet's alongside Tartine's Valrhona chocolate cake.

What you want, baby I got it. Aretha Franklin, Queen of Soul, isn't a client, although years ago nobody could take it to the bridge any better. In a nutshell, *Mr. Haute Coiffure* might very well indeed be all about respect — mind, body, and if you are one believer, spirit as well.

✝

✝

FOREWORD

Sensitive subject, concerning a bastard's birth name. Jean, my mother, wasn't yet divorced from her physically and emotionally abusive, good-for-nothing then-husband; he wasn't my father — mine had his own separate unpleasant issues.

Didn't get an opportunity to see my original birth certificate; the name appearing now wasn't what appeared before tender age eight. Today, legally, I'm Gerard James Schiavo, bearing my biological father's surname.

A side moot jotting will brief you: *Schiavo*, heard or read by any fluent Italian speaker, translates into *slave*. Its Latin origin defines further shedding — *ciao* within *Schiavo*, the root translation means at your service; every Italian uses that word's form delivering hellos and goodbyes. Perfect last name for the hairstylist — *hello, at your service* — spending a career designing my clientele's hair; this writer, however, contracted another moniker more fitting.

Googling "Jehr" instantly locates me; entering "Schiavo" is unnecessary. Since 1977 I am Jehr Schiavo, in some circles known as a celebrated hairstylist. The name Jehr was conceived in beauty school at eighteen selecting letters from Gerard James Schiavo. Later, *Allure* magazine wrote of one-name hairstylists — myself this article's lead, charging $1000 per cut.

I started writing in 2008, borrowing Jean's maiden name, signing my work *Gerard Saint D'Angelo*. Saint wasn't abbreviated St., dual abbreviation for enormous virtuosity and street — the latter an epitome of who I am, having appreciable aspirations — but "Gerard Street D'Angelo" doesn't resonate, does it?

Manuscripts I write begin stating the following: *by Jehr Schiavo writing as Gerard Saint D'Angelo*. The hairstylist of forty years is not this author spilling out line after lines, night and day, months into years.

✝

BY JEHR SCHIAVO
WRITING AS GERARD SAINT D'ANGELO

✝

PREFACE

Every once in awhile we'll catch a professional athlete making his quite intimate sign of the cross before going up at bat, perhaps bloodied fighters facing their menacing opponent within that ring; so too shall football players acknowledging God likewise, though such chaos on NFL turf — alongside cumbersome upper-body uniform and helmet surely diverting visible attention from any cross-signing — recognizing faith: "please help my performance be its best while keeping me injury-free."

There's common perception on-camera game-time that beside faith, courage will also stand in front, as staring down a major league pitcher's ninety-three-mile-an-hour fastball, or suffering any testosterone-filled ultimate fighter's blistering right hook, for all one knows his roundhouse kick to this challenger's temple — last but not least, several two-hundred-and-ninety pounds of defensive muscle leveling their offending team's wide receiver throughout four relentless quarters. I'm no star athlete, yet sense a direct connection when grown men, macho as they're made, deliver without speaking their crossing's reverence, "it is not me alone."

ESPN crews aren't anywhere around here lighting this desk; sound engineers appear nowhere in sight, cameramen neither — whether I'm wearing underwear, robe, or t-shirt and trousers doesn't really matter, should it? I don't recall at what age I'd been taught, but guess about four years old, learned praying, "In the name of the Father, Son, and Holy Ghost." Life be as it may, I began disbelieving faith upon thirteen, while displaying a faux veneer for courage. After two horrible wayward decades I altered fractionally this opener toward innermost thought, "In the name of the Father, Son, and Holy Spirit." Using the word "ghost" in youth distracted me prior to prayer — inevitably comic book character Casper and his apparition's friendly, comical personality crept inside, minimising whatever sacred introspection that I (an especially mischievous junior hellion) had, requiring tremendous forgiveness of countless daily transgressions. Any opportunity to achieve honest-to-God beatification long ago slipped right by me; living my life faultlessly won't ever happen. Suffice it to say, without courage and faith I'd be better off dust.

✝

BY JEHR SCHIAVO
WRITING AS GERARD SAINT D'ANGELO

BY JEHR SCHIAVO
WRITING AS GERARD SAINT D'ANGELO

✝

THE KIDS

Most every child I've ever seen exhibits a beautiful head
of hair; count on kids, though, at times to have goofy cuts
— they just won't sit still, even in romper room kiddie
salons. There is an endearing quality really, concerning
wee ones with botched haircuts, often overshadowed by
his or her striking personality. Inevitably, this child's locks
exude healthy vibrancy, winning above any homemade
bowl cut, or perhaps their own handiwork, completed
when no one had been looking, not even themself.

Freedom by such innocent self-expression begins
early and in far fewer than we might imagine among
many typical children. Harmless, quite frankly — yes,
their negligible mishap style can be an eyesore for that
particular family holiday portrait or school year photo,
causing temporary parental embarrassment walking
together down the grocery store aisle. Fact remains,
while our creative youngster may very well be sporting an
obviously haphazard kitchen scissors done-it-themself
independent moment, their hair itself, by its splendid

texture, nine out of ten times appears in far better condition than too many adults'.

For those grooming miniature beauty pageant hopefuls, artificially fussed upon by age three as grown-up icons, chances are extremely high, regrettably so, that Little Miss Wherever-She's-From lost a certain quality present in other kids' natural unchanged hair's state, likely replaced with damaged tresses similar to adults who've manipulated their hairstyles by heat, possibly chemicals, unsuitably, however, probably both.

At approximately the magic age of twelve Mom's styling products and tools suddenly start to disappear, ending up in her daughter's hands. Not long thereafter, this snowballs in great numbers: their household blow dryers, curling and flat irons, mousses, gels, curl enhancers, heat protectors, hairsprays, round roller brushes, alongside any other items which force hair to do what it usually refuses — temporarily cooperating into preconceived notions. Our novice could take thirty, sometimes ninety, minutes applying those terribly unnecessary lotions and potions before blow drying, then flat ironing, some days finishing using a curling iron; she inspects her struggle, when on occasion — might also happen to Mom — they'll separately go right back into the shower full of frustration, shampooing, conditioning another round, absurdly reasoning it came out unsatisfactory their first attempt at perfection (life ain't perfect either, honey).

As the personal identity experimental process seduces us, we succumb to those professionals providing various services: a hairstylist, whose input is usually based primarily upon their income, and our local beauty supply store employees, who also seldom have regard for what customers apply over virgin or previously chemically treated hair.

✝

✝

T. Rex

Personal testimony here: in a twenty-seven month
span, from the freshman hours studying cosmetology
onto attaining one highly sought-after stylist position
at Vidal Sassoon, after completing their arduous year-
long apprenticeship program, I made these ridiculous
major alterations to my own unprocessed hair. Permed it,
disliked that, then straightened what had originally been
gentle waves at shorter lengths to soft curls, growing
longer, normal southern Italian hair. Displeased by this
one-hundred-eighty-degree texture transformation,
I eventually dove into color, bleaching my once again
virgin, inch-long dark brown hair completely out to
white, then dying it six weeks later Elvis jet blue-black.

Granted, as any beauty college student can tell you,
practicing procedures on doll heads with yak hair will
quickly become rather humdrum. Not every walk-
in patron is always enthusiastic to allow freshmen
carte blanche. Regular beauty school clients routinely
telephone, scheduling appointments how anyone else

should, requesting senior students — a much safer choice, my friends.

While senior students beyond our closed-off, glassed-in freshman room waited for their next appointments — maybe already working on this particular school's prevalent patron, an elderly retired woman — we attacked each other's hair during the grueling initial four-hundred-hour tenderfoot segment. Class started out, as I recall, close to a dozen, dropping census by over half that in those early months before being permitted outside the newcomers' glass cage enclosure. Instantly this whole experimental world was our oyster, as the school chemical dispensary now became completely accessible — cinnamon hair Monday, blonde Wednesday, blue on Friday.

It may be of interest: myself and two other men comprised that entire student body's straight male population. Why would this scale-tipping gay-men-to-straight-male hairstylist ratio have any merit whatsoever?— it shouldn't, although a huge factor, not only from experience during sixteen hundred hours attending cosmetology school, but another perspective, observing behind the scenes, as an outsider these four decades within my profession.

Young girls enjoy playing dress up, as can boys their age, with a naïve proclivity favoring his own sex. Throw into this flamboyant mix pop culture's gender-bending formative era with glam rock's onslaught by His High Priest or Priestess of Androgynous *Ch-ch-changes*, David

Bowie. The early to late 70s were that explosive phase — glitter's New York Dolls morphed into punk rock's Ramones, while disco's flagship Studio 54 paved way for rap's upcomers, Sugarhill Gang and Grandmaster Flash. In beauty college especially, if you didn't shape your eyebrows you'd stick out like a drag queen inside some busy Bakersfield truck stop bathroom. Anyway, why not — Freddy Mercury definitely waxed, Mick Jagger pushed his feminine image too, right beyond the edge. Deloux School of Cosmetology for me acted through its chemical lab an excellent daytime rock 'n' roll backstage — testing procedures on ourselves exclusively, surely not our frail elderly regulars. At my eighteenth year, peer pressure overwhelmed me being the minority; confinment weeks on end finally took its toll with young Mr. Haute Coiffure's hair, eyebrows, and nails. That human guinea pig beauty experimentation could very well be labeled "finding yourself" by manner of cosmetology school disasters.

✝

BY JEHR SCHIAVO
WRITING AS GERARD SAINT D'ANGELO

✝

SF (Once Upon A Time)✝

Up above Grant Avenue between Geary and O'Farrell
in San Francisco was Sassoon's chemical department,
adjacent to their men's barbershop. Downstairs at ground
level, reception and client changing rooms, leading
toward its wide-open cutting area, plenty of it: twenty
styling chairs, not including five shampoo basins, hidden
behind the back bar's white cabinetry, exposing enough
space that anyone curious could observe comings or
goings about upstairs.

At that time I'd been so engaged shampooing sixteen
heads, maybe more, on a daily basis, I hadn't actually
given thought to what clever design it was situating this
shampoo area facing the salon's only stairway. Elegant
then, and would be presently, most every vertical wall
was painted a truffle cocoa powder brown, which created

✝ I'll almost certainly skip between different intervals throughout this satirical view
of the beauty industry, foreseeably estimating exact dates — can't refer to a journal, I
haven't ever consistently kept one. Long-term memories appear veiled, but absolutely
connected; my story is reliable, though not linear.

an effect of mystery, specifically within that center-rear stairwell.

During any slammin' day one hundred sixty clients could be shampooed and conditioned by ten ruthless competitive assistants, serving their two assigned stylists on a six-week rotation. A question industry mogul Sassoon perhaps demanded of the interior design firm creating that Grant Avenue space: "How can my business increase by doubling each day's one hundred sixty-client maximum load into three hundred twenty clients?" Gifted interior genius perhaps probed, "What else will your salon offer clients other than precision haircuts?" By the 1970s' latter half, fifteen years then running strong in North America, Vidal no doubt shed light on those lucrative point-of-sale purchases, brought by urging chemical service, responding to his interior designer: "color, tints, highlights, lowlights, perms, body waves, and relaxers."

In general people are curious; being snoopy is innate for most. We'll also believe a desire that what someone other than ourselves has should be ours too — though odds are reasonably high, we don't absolutely require that item not currently in our possession. When children behave in similar fashion, responsible parents balance their child's behavior, shun thinking they're only being kids, instead encouraging, "Buffy, give Miffy her mouse back, it's not yours."

Precisely how many clients I shampooed on Grant Avenue throughout that Sassoon apprenticeship

program would be mere estimation — ballparking
thousands, actually upward for accuracy, but rounding
down realistically to three thousand. Practically each
client I ever shampooed and conditioned, alongside
nearly all other patrons, overhearing adjoining back
bar conversation inquired, "What's upstairs?" While
massaging my stylist's robed client's worldly cares
momentarily aside with frothy almond-scented bubbles,
she'd as expected close her weary eyes, wondering what
fabulous treatments might be discovered climbing that
rich chocolate stairwell, watching another set of footsteps
sound their departing appearance, having one other
service she herself may have lacked — missing out on
ravishing color, tint applied from two-ounce tubes, third-
distillation coal tar blended with, at best, twenty-volume
peroxide, right upstairs.

Much too frequently we'll do just about anything to
project ourselves as our absolute favorite celebrities — those
we may not necessarily envy, but who became the single
most special character seen on television, film or magazine
covers; for these individuals shy of self-confidence,
this sadly is their primary flaw in personal beauty.

Typical of many salons there comes this day: an entire
staff room will be filled with stylists anxiously waiting —
at extremely slow periods, minutes dragging into hours,
newspapers having been separated from their neatly folded
sections, crossword puzzles completed, personal phone
calls made, pastries, breakfast sandwiches, later Chow
Mein eaten, coffee maker on its umpteenth pot, and while

21

law still permitted in 1977, ashtrays teemed by chain-smoking nervous commission employees' cigarette butts.

Strange gathering, these colleagues, each stylist directly competing against one another's bigger paycheck — shallow statement, although for the most part, bragging rights took place returning from lunch breaks carrying top-name designer shopping bags. Vidal Sassoon, in the heartbeat of San Francisco's fashionable Union Square, couldn't have been a more convenient location for our busier, but shopaholic, stylists. If I'm not mistaken certain personalities purchased looks of that immediate trend, showed it off for approval in our staff room, and returned those ostentatious garments within minutes following a jealous gang's disapproval; moreover, their paycheck hadn't to-date afforded such lavish fads — not that this wasn't the killer piece, expressly, assuming it were.

✝

✝

BECOMING BLONDE

Who's wearing what today? The morning decision burden weighed heavy on me back then, becoming a Sassoon-promoted stylist from lowly assistant. I'd gone positively bonkers shortly following twelve-noon's shopping spree parade. Twenty-year-old Mr. Haute Coiffure thought, what's free of charge which would make an unequivocal bold statement? I mosied up from the staff room basement, cruised reception, verbally blocking out a few hours that midweek day — seemed awfully slow anyway — disappearing up our scrumptious chocolate stairwell.

Me, these days, dependable as they come — for what purpose should I replace names of those guilty individuals? A considerable distance in time shielding them; now some infelicitous comments about Lori, our senior colorist on Grant Avenue. I won't flatter myself replying yes, telling you nor anyone inquiring, "Had Lori been solely flirtatious with yourself, or was she purely craving male attention wherever her eyes landed?"

Whoever lied, saying gentlemen don't ever kiss and tell, probably didn't fully understand there are certain circumstances, those exceptions; why, you're thinking — allow an explanation.

Before that first year's humiliating assistant experience was complete, we'd previously been separated by two department floors — myself then occasionally escorting a client to color, or Lori personally delivering clients downstairs, receiving my designated stylist's instructions for an apprentice blow dry. She'd not yet touched me — okay, I'm stretching matters, admissibly once, while completely polluted during the salon manager Thomas' Polish wedding reception at St. Dominic's Catholic Church.

Requesting my hair be bleached out white shouldn't have been an issue, I figured; it wasn't. Lori pointed me straight toward the color department's rack containing brown robes, ordering, "Go ahead, take off your shirt, put on one of those." Thought, oh man, this is gonna be great fun; at last I'm an equal, no more dinking around with me, who cares how long it takes to strip my hair.

Seated on a plush caramel-brown hydraulic styling chair, gazing into one of the empty barbershop's tubular chrome-framed mirrors, I waited as Lori concocted those proper chemical ingredients inside her color department's dispensary. An entire second floor to ourselves; only two of the half-dozen or so barber chairs were ever occupied, tucked aside within a spacious winged alcove. Lori appeared holding a

plastic translucent martini-shaped color bowl, beige
surgical rubber gloves, and black applicator brush. Soon
as she placed those items on an available waist-high
metal rolling tray, presently at my nose height, a bizarre
sensation began to occur. Habañero peppers have an
ability to clear up clogged sinuses; they'll make us quickly
break out in a feverish sweat — not much of anything
can douse this fire we set ablaze inside our mouth. Her
concoction seemed delightfully appetizing — you'd just
want to ingest spoonful after spoonfuls, mouth-watering
as clotted cream — however, thoroughly commanded
a noxious odor. Any foreign matter lodged inside my
nasal cavity instantly vanished, obliterated — much the
same effect wasabi, spicy curry, or serrano peppers have,
although I hadn't tasted Lori's private bleach reserve,
simply whiffed it inches away.

   Us, those responsible, speak out, remaining
accountable for our every action. Hear me, not only
should Lori take blame, I'll assume more than partial
fault; there, I said it — I'm half culpable by allowing
what no level-headed person should've let happen. Even
if I hadn't studied how powerful bleach was after being
applied to hair in beauty college, any imbecile who didn't
would have realized just from the toxic smell alone that
a horrible result could very well be possible. The Food
Network's Anne Burrell along with Guy Fieri are two
people playing with fire beyond their kitchen cooktops,
trading hair for moussed cotton candy and baby chick
fuzz, respectively.

In fairness, I'm not suggesting if the stylist who colors your hair relays how safe or natural their salon products are, you should dare investigate; prodding them to eat one spoonful before application can bear a distinct confrontational demeanor. Why not casually ask if he or she will give yourself the teeniest tiny lick first, check and see; by this manner, they'll believe trusting their word plays a major factor. Any salon, beauty store, or health food grocer selling so-called organic and natural hair color should also stock on their establishment's shelves cans of gelatinous Spam. Neither hair dye nor processed meat are chemical-free; don't believe me, go buy the Brooklyn Bridge.

This faux platinum recipient observed dark brown hair going through several lighter tones during my bleach pack's initial hour, resting directly on the scalp as well — impossible to avoid, we should talk about that. Temperature felt cool, then began tingling, practically rejuvenating, as the skin and follicles started tightening; all of a sudden, almost in an instant (didn't even switch slowly to warm) my scalp within seconds burst into virtual flames.

"When's this stuff coming off Lori, where are we now?"

"Is your head getting hot?— don't worry, you'll be alright, besides it's only come up pale yellow so far; if Marilyn handled it, so can you."

Meantime, Lori adjusted three heat lamps: one pointing directly toward the back of my head, two facing each side, all of them shining partially on top. When those lamps glowing from their orange flood-shaped bulbs were set in place, my whole scalp seemingly exploded into molten lava — stunning shade, a bright meteor ball of flames starting at the shoulders. Applied heat speeds up the chemical process — in this case, stubborn hair unwilling to turn white; today your preferred salon has their marginally updated robotic model.

Further insulting my narrow threshold for pain, Lori joked, saying Marilyn Monroe continued icing her nether regions days after applying bleach, matching the color above. What felt like hours later — don't recall for sure — became deliriously amiss after an unspecified period frying by beauty chemicals, centimeters from my brain — in spite of which I can still hear her assistant Atis, conducting his quick strand test with a nervous chuckle, blurting, "Uh oh, I better get Lori." That's the vote of confidence nobody wants — not anyone hoping to emulate Marilyn Monroe nor impressionable me, secretly wishing I could quasi-modify Lou Reed's character during his legendary *Sally Can't Dance* tour.[†]

Biting my laced tongue not only heightened Lori's shocked state of paranoia rinsing her colleague's hair, but also Atis' inspection over the shampoo basin. Both Lori's and Atis' petrified faces peered down at my

---

[†] Amazing, I haven't cursed so far, promised myself there would be no justification uttering flagrant profanity, could deter extremely modest sorts interested by what's written across these pages. I've concluded sufficient vulgarity in five other manuscripts, thereby fully compensating for an absence of foul language from beginning to end inside this book.

soaked yet invisible hair, as if neither had ever witnessed such a cataclysmic feat in their combined professional careers. By touch, my wet opaque hair felt similar to that of drenched down goose feathers; gently pulled for an elasticity test, mine shredded apart, as if picking at today's catch — Dungeness crab.

✢

✝

Le Coiffeur

During these last several years I've exerted spare
energy eliminating worldly possessions. I got rid of
stuff which felt an overabundance; when it came right
down to what was significant or necessary, hardly a great
quantity remains. If such a point should arise within
these confines of pertinence concerned, I'll manage
what's possible describing lightening life inside *Mr. Haute
Coiffure*. For the present, I'm sure briefly, there is a single
item I've recently regretted having not made my keepers
pile. Once a favorite: an ancient, hardbound book about
hair — shouldn't have been gifted to another, although
I did. When I age and lose faculties, wouldn't matter
in any case, whether nearby or wherever this treasure
happens to then be.

What vital information that frayed and yellowed gem
contained, I've stored in my mind's personal cloud. Of
the book's countless illustrations, I can still remember
this specific image, a quarter-page-size sketch of Her
Majesty's (don't know who in particular) — French,

German, Italian, perchance Spanish — their royal citadel's hairdresser. Centuries so long ago, those pictured could be seen wearing elfin slip-on ankle boots — castle slippers, if you will. Since her 1953 coronation Queen Elizabeth II refuses to change hairstyles. Quite possibly the very same hairdresser and protégé have been but only a stone's toss, near her dressing area ever since.

Unless, of course, you are that extremely prosperous figure guiding a publicly traded company, hiring your own private hairstylist twenty-four-seven-three-six-five, this personal luxury would be unquestionably difficult to budget — not for Hillary Clinton nor Carly Fiorina.

In the olden days this merry bunch primping over an immediate royal family might've been paid by soup and bread. These days a handful of hairstylists charge ludicrous fees — that trend inadvertently brought up during my February 2001 interview for *Allure* magazine.

Across more than the Americas, cropping up quicker than this earth can rotate, marks property leased to well-known beauty brand names; yet increasingly, beauticians numbering millions no one will ever hear about — many of whom shouldn't have bothered wasting tuition attending cosmetology school — open salons every day. Complete urban blocks in big cities — perfectly cute smaller towns, too — lined with hair salons, estheticians, and the excessively rampant Vietnamese mani-pedi salon. Word must've gotten out, flood gates unlocked: clock in 1,600 beauty college hours, be present ten months without missing a single day, and any quickie online GED high school graduate may swiftly earn six figures yearly.

Seldom will any stylist remain under the salon owner's thumb — nor should they, basically working for peanuts. At a commission rate of fifty percent — lower, actually — owners devised an untenable sliding-scale wage system; incidentally most salons can't provide substantial foot traffic from walk-in trade to support their famished stylists. Subtract another double-digit percentage, allocated toward the Internal Revenue Service and other frequent outrageous demands: all too often an employee must purchase their salon's personalized business cards, also pay for mandatory health insurance; commissioned hairstylists receive paychecks which commonly infuriate them.

If stylists you've met with have shown a persistent off-putting attitude, but snuck in comments regarding their mind-blowing nightlife during that period following your last appointment, here, you're glimpsing why. Detesting one's position is a tremendously meaningful issue. Clients' hair suffers when their stylist lacks focus — possibly they'd been carousing way too late prior to those next-day appointments, not out of the question, in acute cases arriving directly from clubbing — then it once again becomes time for an improved, newer salon.

Second among three salon business models, much to the chagrin of any shrewd entrepreneurial owner, are those salons renting chairs on a monthly basis. These establishments rake in every dollar from each client's retail point-of-sale purchase; however, that's that, finito, whatever services rendered through this owner's renter is income exclusive to the stylist.

Thriving companies report growth: steadfast, equally-matched increments over decades, as Costco does, or this global phenomenon growing at instantaneous supersonic measures, those renowned high-level tech giants. Chair rentals most certainly provide a better deal for the stylist than previous employment elsewhere, having been gouged by commission-based salon owners.

Purely from a financial standpoint, any chair rental salon is inevitably capped by the square feet for chairs; flat, completely void of significant gain unless an owner derives pleasure managing egocentric personalities or gets kicks playing landlord. What monetary control this salon type doesn't have renting chairs is then compensated by the owner's enormous array of available beauty products; each stylist possibly or may not be permitted a fractional pittance in percentage from their clients' retail purchases.

Simultaneously tempers ignite among stylists who've suddenly aligned themselves in opposition against the evil salon owners. Renters have much more leverage than commissioned employees. Motivated stylists assuming business risk work through these ranks until they themselves obtain enough savings to open their own establishments. Who hasn't heard those stories about walkouts, when an entire salon of stylists pack up tools and Rolodexes, scheduling clients at home before beauty equipment they've leased is installed, renting a vacant storefront across the street from where they'd been insulted — given one measly percent from their clients' retail product sales, thereby concluding category three.

If we're aware, even plagued by obscure sensitivity, we notice thick tension throughout salons everywhere. It feels plain uncomfortable; most clients simply can't wait to get out of there, but they continue returning time and again because hair grows, perhaps more frequently than preferred. Merciless cycle from any client's perspective — their stylist, along with the salon owner, is in many respects a constant revolving door to all affected parties. Stylists might jump ship next week by reason of throat-cutting and back-stabbing today; however, salon connivers shall forever persist, still categorizing their profession as the "beauty industry," an ugly business cranking out our utmost important adornment.

✝

✢

EXEMPTION

Over the past four decades, I prevail a radical beauty thinker, humbled by that process which has afforded me accolades, reached through means on my terms, staying to this day grateful and evermore. Structured walls inside any dysfunctional salon were outside the domain of satisfaction; I shun the beauty industry, one shamelessly riddled by greed, displaying petty integrity, if any at all.

Rolling along thus far you and I are both settled, there's two methods of handling situations, another mainstream strategy or one hundred eighty degree conflicting extreme. "Your hair will fall out if it's chemically treated," not true. I'm polemic at heart; counteracted by means of an artistic mind, high contrast viewing most every life aspect, for me unadulterated — opposition though, often outright turbulent.

✢

✝

Mountains

Addicted overweight human cherubs gorge — oh God,
I almost wrote "pig out," but stopped, reminding myself
how crude that would be. Making conscious but blurred
decisions, poisoning themselves, drug fiends and drunks,
they pig out — seems hardly ill-mannered, yet exposes
my empathy's bias; intellectual ability is a terrible
waste. Vain folks have difficulty prying themselves from
mirrors, expressing arrogant pretension in gory intricacy
concerning plastic surgery procedures they recently had
done, including how magnificently the imminent future
modifications shall enhance their superior beauty.

I've been downright irresponsible abusing: food,
drugs, alcohol, and an overindulgence of self-absorption,
acting these four character traits throughout different
spells. I've refused to prevent junk food from entering
my mouth, cookies mostly, age eight until thirteen,
stopped that addiction almost immediately — no really,
practically overnight — favoring instead liquor and
drugs; added vanity upon turning sixteen, embarrasingly

enough continued obsessing over appearances when alopecia proved myself flawed by about twenty-eight years old; maturing into life's realistic conditions finally at thirty-three. By what exorbitant price did this set me back — well, I'll require lost receipts describing years abusing sweets; Budweiser, Remy Martin; cigarettes; pot; diving into a pure degenerative lifestyle, consuming every form of mood-elevating upper, downer, hallucinogen, opiate; eventually worshipping snowflake-fluffy cocaine, while booking weekly facials, biannual peelings, microdermabrasions, manicures and pedicures, essentially attempting to clean up the despicable mess I'd created. Unfortunately, all such expenses were obviously flushed down the toilet, figuratively and literally. Luck along with prayers and perseverance forced my feet onto an alternate route, ultimately replenishing a squandered quarter century's personal financial solvency.

Here's the kicker: what doesn't grow on trees (as I posit currency's cotton does) is this rare natural quality which sadly eludes a high degree of mortals, breathing life — peacefully content, sincerely pleased illuminating wellness inside ourselves.

Easy and painless, not necessarily superb medicine. At age eight began weekends on my own; Mom bussed to work by sunrise, delayed many evenings working overtime, returned home after dark in a thirteen-plus-hour mood. Jean overindulged me with sweets, in my estimation compensating for her absence; she couldn't buy them fast enough. I jiggled walking anywhere two years later, stuffing my face while watching television, both before and after school. Exact recipe for a youth's setback, scholastically and socially. Ah, that then-recently discovered thrill, self-anesthetizing. I affiliated myself with any similar juvenile delinquents, usually older and more advanced in the realm of foolery. Retracing steps which led nowhere was half the battle. First, choosing health's well-being, rather than hiding behind addictions, maintaining this dauntless pursuit beyond incisive assessment with due diligence (psychotherapist not included), should also provide others with positive benefits. Frivolous me, hadn't been legitimately prepared by eight years old.[+][‡]

[+] My opinion determined redundancy causes mild nausea within myself, repeating twice and again, then additional conveyances as though, if it were me guilty being charged, I've an imagination bordered by restricted expanse or kind of a lazy sort. Rewriting that which I already wrote earlier isn't a defect I'm willing to assume accountability for. Pardon me; I'm a bit concerned with the topic at hand, making reference to my own quotes, passages or complete wordage, front cover throughout this book's final page.

[‡] Several years ago I posted a piece online called "Patron Etiquette," opting not to paraphrase said article here or virtually cheat on this body's work by insertion, when convenient if inclined, compare differences between conventional salon mechanics and mine transformed into reality, written with the impression of intimation. Perhaps there could have been an auxiliary format communicating what I'd hope to bring forth, speaking in that possibility of how dull, moderate or drastic we build the framework for client and stylist suitability, hence a successful relationship.

✝

Ears Put to Use

An extensive chunk of my styling career demanded listening — still does, I'll hear thorough volumes. Where curricular education failed to teach formally, paying close attention has been this outcast's graduate program, standing alongside most chat-friendly patrons seated for Jehrcuts, less that half-million-dollar Ph.D. loan.

Personal client stories express variations, although their common denominator fits almost perfectly into anticipated molds — those modes of behavior strictly characterized by living above or below expectations and standards — yet great numbers seldom ever genuinely alter much positive life-changing substance within themselves, other than an occasional different hairstyle.

So many clients are under the misconception that a hairstylist can make them happy. Venturing out on a delicate limb presently, in all plausibility your hairstylist lives with perplexities you wouldn't want to know they have. A client will confide, make confessions, deeply reflecting concerns which shaped life while the trusted stylist attends their crowning glory. Too close for comfort, a fragile dichotomy, addressing our client's appearance during intimate detailed conversation; this twisted connotation invariably translates into, at that immediate moment, their new hairstyle — an expeditious answer to life's myriad of challenges.

Whether hairstylists recognize it or not, they're essentially wizards of an unspoken mutual agreement, "You're going to fix me by the time our appointment is over, correct?"

"Absolutely, okay sweetie, how about a few highlights, we'll disguise your gray, it'll have you feeling and looking fifteen years younger."

An entire appointment, she spills her delicate guts, telling the stylist what misery she'd recently gone through — left for a younger woman, being awarded custody of their children following divorce. One may speculate why any astute woman should ever select male sashay as her chief beauty advisor and confidant, concluding that he understands men intimately, conveniently decorates hair, and does not threaten women. If choosing another, the female stylist, sharing identical commissary, this can frequently deflate that sympathy she'd hoped for when scheduling an appointment.

✝

⚜

LIARS AND LIES

I'll preface this next part with an unfeigned apology
sent to any little boy who long ago insisted upon whiling
the hours away playing with someone else's Barbie or
whose inappropriate parents broke down, caved in, even
encouraged his very own toy doll. If your grandfather,
father, son, brother, uncle, male cousin or best non-
boyfriend found amusement giving Barbie an updo
by age four, then twenty-five years later opened and
operates his salon, it's definitely reasonable some could
be perturbed, believing I've unfairly singled out, isolating
the beauty industry's predominate workforce — not to
say some heterosexual hairstylists aren't ever at fault,
either. I have, though, a sensible peek at exploitation
waged against faithful clients.

Does your hair, makeup and nails have a slight
resemblance to Barbie or another iconic plastic doll you've
seen? Can you run an open hand fingering through your
hair without it feeling accurately, if not closely, similar to
poor Barbie's locks, unhealthy and completely synthetic?

What any grandfather, father, son, brother, uncle, male cousin or best non-boyfriend have intimate aim for is his, perhaps her, transgender rightful prerogative. When it became evident by inordinate instances that male sashay's fundamental beauty premise had adverse client consequences, specifically on women's hair, this eventually brought to light an issue Mr. Haute Coiffure should no longer find honorable ignoring.

Many will falsely ascertain I'm closed-minded, even homophobic, criticizing the content they've interpreted thus far — exclaiming it's hardly rhetorical, refusing to read my books and articles ever again. Three cheers, hooray for us, surely as time ticks on, so shall those satisfied who continue to read this book; comprehending these chapters may indeed change your hair, improving remarkably, though why halt there?

Frustrating as it is, believe the inevitable: no set of highlights can ever be duplicated, an especially big problem if you happen to have fallen madly in love with a particular favored appointment's results. An accomplished colorist tediously weaves hair to be colored before applying tint or bleach, placing that specified meticulous amount onto foil, neatly creasing those aluminium squares for processing. No accomplished colorist will ever again be able to place that exact, previously specified tedious amount of colored hair onto foil for processing. Unfortunately, each future appointment from then forward finds more hair which wasn't colored prior, becoming lighter too. Eventually, the whole head is no longer its original intention of sun-kissed highlights, but rather dull, drab, and one-dimensional — seemingly having received a single-process tint, possessing that common, typical salon synthetic appearance suffering brittle texture, which (making matters worse) can only be cosmetically remedied by blow drying, possibly flat ironing stick-straight, or using curling irons to create voluptuous, crispy barrel curls. Adding insult to injury, an accomplished savvy colorist will always later introduce lowlights, applying darker tints, attempting counterbalance for a bleached-out, over-processed look.

This chemical money pit doesn't ever end, yet it's not an amusement park where the roller coaster automatically stops. You're either brave understanding highlights are a salon's expensive wild ride starting out, telling yourself when to call it quits or simply say no off the bat; getting hair back into its natural state can take what will feel like an eternity.

No accomplished savvy colorist jeopardizes income, refusing application of a client's subsequent chemical service because their hair had become trashed due to his or her astounding achievements.

Another revealing actuality: hair is a direct link to our state of mind, self-esteem, how we place ourselves on the existence totem pole. Clients who arrived for their very first consultation with damaged, functionally impaired tresses — short, mid, or long lengths — had an air about them which reflected that persona they projected, having at that point previously worn only permanent bad hair days.

Remarkable how chic, effortless, healthy, sustainable hair can look and feel. Receiving the proper cut followed by prescription for homecare lends tremendous enhancement to this once unassured client — their psyche bursting afterward with an undivided, lately found confidence in themself and life.

Do you reckon we've ditched this trail of any overly defensive critics? I've a covert acknowledgment, I didn't actually welcome their cattiness anyway; most realize sly haters can't survive without vindictiveness.

Of an industry ruled by a gay cartel, remaining heterosexual creates apparent obstacles. In any other business environment, blatant discriminatory ridicule isn't condoned; elsewhere, such treatment would be commonly referred to as sexual harassment. Me, fifty-seven upon manuscript's completion — -eight at publication — my overall physical tone ain't what it used to be. If I, by deserved reason, had been sentenced to any maximum correctional facility in my twenties, thirties, or early forties, this might've been cause for due anxiety; since I'm further seasoned than fifty years old, walking within some prison yard or inside a beauty salon doesn't actually matter, does it — nobody's whistling at me in either venue today.

Out of respect — homage, one might say — for those elite few, world-class, five-star flaming hairdressers, prior to the early 1960s, they were regularly addressed, *Mister*

43

Such and So. Who had been the prominent hairdressers expecting this ceremonious formality I'll not list; my educated belief, most were gay — who needs uncalled-for headaches stemming from lawsuits?

I desired an indisputable benevolent title, one which would age well long after I'm not around, a parody coined of an industry often wrongfully doubting me — who, too, in this business, could wisely embrace this adversary. Mr. Haute Coiffure, steady at the helm, bedewing that little boy's fire growing up — soon otherwise misleading women by treating their female clientele's beauty vaguely different than a life-size Barbie.

✝

BY JEHR SCHIAVO
WRITING AS GERARD SAINT D'ANGELO

✝

MOM, NO APPLE PIE

I brushed Jean's hair late on Thursday afternoon at
Mercy Hospital, a day before her unsuccessful surgery
thirteen years ago this December 2016. She was seventy-
nine; sorrow recognizes I often feel robbed having her
big-hearted voice for only forty-five nurturing years.
Staying perfectly explicit, Mom hadn't planned on
becoming pregnant in 1957 by any means; unaware of
his marital status, she astonished my alcoholic father
informing him about her pregnancy, whereupon he stuck
out one cowardly hand, delivered a chilly "good luck,"
turned away, and proceeded straight back home to an
unsuspecting betrayed wife. Not yet visibly showing, Jean
then carried me, pressing forward by herself, a decidedly
proud, tough, beautiful woman.

Four years later, following Jean single-handedly
raising me from birth, mini Master Haute Coiffure
took it upon himself to remain nearby her any moments
possible, between Mom's two full-time Ozone Park, New
York jobs: days as a factory piecework seamstress, nights

45

waitressing at the Americana Lanes Coffee Shop. Proud, tough while beautiful, thoroughly Sicilian, Jean in those days was hardly patient; her composure gradually evolved through life, though by the time I turned five, getting knocked around meant she cared for me before leaving to work or recently having returned home. I missed her; she'd been gone from seven in the morning through that midnight, with a ninety-minute exception, racing to fix dinner at four-thirty, then hurrying herself into an evening's all-white waitress uniform.

I wasn't typically received well in our apartment's small kitchen until Mom finished cooking; sure, maybe I'd sneak a look smelling from the doorway, although with that wooden spaghetti spoon at close range, better to keep out of Jean's way.

An Italian family meal is a near religious experience — stuffed mushrooms, sometimes artichokes, manicotti, every so often veal scallopini or eggplant parmesan, then again grilled fennel sausage and peppers always satisfy; it's our sacred moment at most any Sicilian table, crusty bread with sesame seeds, small chunks in hand, broken off the daily loaf, lively conversation while chewing. Some Italians, we can finagle both together at once like an elite ventriloquist will; I can't remember blood relatives ever disciplining, "Don't talk with your mouth full."

If I hadn't behaved appropriately during Jean's working hours, trouble in my case transferred into consequence, beside receiving her cold shoulder. Vandalizing, fighting, cursing, stealing — alongside their

dearest ally, the equivocator — were habitually displayed
silently screaming out, "give me attention right this
second." On a rare off chance that somehow Jean hadn't
discovered my serious offenses or miraculously someway
had inexplicably gone any day blameworthy-free, I
received the special tenderness she tightly guarded —
showing affection, permitting me close to her side.

Mom was in my childhood mind as I'll endlessly recall,
a brunette goddess, her face creamy smooth, having
shapely lips, both eyes holding loving stories — if there
were only more hours in our day. Jeanette, my precious
wife, is both aware and pleased Jean was young Master
Haute Coiffure's first love. Mom's eyesight at seventy
years old had been diagnosed with macular degeneration.
Legally blind, Mom learned without sight through a
heightened sense of touch; eight years later Jeanette felt
Jean's hands cradle her cheeks upon meeting each other;
an only son found beauty truly matched — passing the
torch, mother to wife.

Jeanette was not in attendance at Mercy Hospital
while I brushed Jean's hair twelve years ago, nor LouLou
our daughter, the spitting image of Jean, then barely
two months old. That hospital wasn't an environment
fitting for a newborn infant nor Mom's agonized likeness
which Jeanette's memory should store. Jeanette hadn't
ever observed me brushing Jean's hair, not while visiting
the ecstatic nonna in San Diego when LouLou was six
weeks old nor Mom and Jeanette's first acquaintance
that previous year, as Jean, without complete vision,

47

prepared favorite dishes of mine, celebrating my forty-fifth birthday.

What mental image Jeanette I'm certain would prefer over visualizing my brushing Jean's hair behind an inclined hospital bed, connected alive by mankind's eerie medical monitors, could be picturing those glorious occasions now fifty-four years ago: age four, standing atop our dinette kitchen chair — Master Haute Coiffure, brush in hand, gently sliding strokes through her Ava Gardner hairstyle before she kissed me goodnight — then rushing off to work.

✝

✝

SAGE ADVICE

Such deprivation, allocating an extra few minutes each day for yourself — worse, waiting until you'll become ancient, so incapacitated, might but a good-natured orderly visit the nursing convalescent room, creating that extra-special moment, doing what you had forever failed to care about, brushing your own hair.

Why so many people neglect themselves, refusing whatever this requires, being altogether mindful when it comes to taking care of ourselves, is probably written within psychology journals which have already been pursued. Let's for now forget about why, agreeing reasons obvious, identifiable or unknown. Human nature doesn't until our mid-thirties start withdrawing, backing away from outside influences, earlier perceived important, maturity then accelerates, shifting toward an unfamiliar deeper journey within.

Mirror on my wall, who's the fairest of them all, though in plain fact, mirrors do indeed pose a delusive smoke screen. Since 1982 no patron of mine has ever sat before a mirror, excluding 1989 through 1991 — however those two brief, particular years really shouldn't count. A justifiable error, signing my pneuma over to Lucifer; I purchased an existing salon merely for the fabulously lush annual cash flow. Good God, I simply couldn't help myself — social influence, those nagging additional outside sources, drive some of us batty.

Clients practically coo while I've brushed their hair before cutting, further expressing, why don't I continue that hour's appointment just using my brush — "Who needs a haircut, you can do this for me all day long." After everything is said and done there's no excuse in failing to brush hair daily. I quite possibly — without question — might have a way with my brush, but certainly didn't invent brushing. From the dawn of acknowledged personal beauty, not long before Cleopatra, toga-clad apothecarists obtained crucial understanding how utterly beneficial brushing hair is.

After explaining the best method for significant results when brushing hair correctly, I'll usually complete my lesson, personalizing it by asking clients, "Hadn't your grandmother ever taught you this same technique?" The resounding answer at nearly every instance is an awakened face, as if a misplaced cozy cashmere sweater had been found one frosty February morning.

Inevitably, grandmothers worldwide possess a vast wealth of information; they'll surprise us, giving unadorned solutions for most circumstances. Providing passage through intimate conversation, from grandmothers to mothers, onto their young daughters and sons, readying this partially toothless child for life often begins sharing similar tales: "When Grandma was a little girl..." Who remembers every inch we're taught, specifically while being lulled to sleep after Mom brushed our hair at night before bed?

Beauty before the mid-twentieth century had been an era punctuated with bygone innocence, black and white movies reigned supreme. She was a mystifying actress, who she'd been were dozens. Jean Harlow, eventually teenage Lauren Bacall — their fastidious directors perched them on set dressed in formal sleeping ensembles, solo at that ornate boudoir's vanity, sitting, brushing her hair, wistfully wondering when Cagney or Bogart would ring.

✝

✛

Brush With Fame

This could be a precarious section I may live to regret. I've a lengthy history shooting from the hip — personally and in business, akin to what within seconds flat should pretty much enormously increase sales through my endorsement; however, neither Mr. Haute Coiffure nor Jehr Schiavo presently reaps profit through Mason Pearson — we have zero affiliation. On the subject of hairbrushes, this current day's finest would be manufactured by Mason Pearson, but I'm seriously tempted to tweak that, having persistent requests for my own refined brush, bearing superior quality.

Right here some may presume that if I were truly clever this would be a grand opportunity to have contractual alignment with Mason Pearson. They began perfecting brushes an astounding one hundred years after the United States Declaration of Independence and too America's Constitution; their solid-founded English company hasn't required expertise by Mr. Haute Coiffure. This is a sprawling, open, and free country, land of terrific entrepreneurial opportunity, having many doors leading into unknown endeavors. If Mason Pearson should continue to disregard my gratis recommendation, I'd confess this could be great impetus moving forward as one of their top competitors.

Perhaps some canny publisher would view enterprise differently, suggesting my hasty business decisions be curtailed, tugging in the straps; besides literature acumen, commercialism is also their forte. Emphasis you'll note, speaking so highly about their classic brush by no stretch of the imagination means I carry any Mason Pearson connection whatsoever; if a professional relationship does develop, this entry shall be deleted before publishment, then rewritten accordingly.

Research internet prices, may the best asking price win; there, now you have it, assurance I've lost my marbles. At $165, each brush far exceeds this book's price, approximately sixteen-and-a-half times' worth; sell one million copies, enough readers order their brushes online, Mason Pearson's profit without doubt should easily surpass any publisher's percentage from my literary work.

If and when any behemoth biotech company scientifically develops a process which can extract while bottling for us custom individualized sebaceous oil in serum form that may be applied to our own hair, Mason Pearson brush sales would then undergo financial suffering. My guess, it's probably a lot more cost-effective shelling out $165 on the brush than buying innumerable two-ounce glass vials of personalized sebaceous oil.

Retailers carrying such a product would be incapable of offering affordable prices, charging at least that exact price of your Mason Pearson purchase.

Different from other brushes, the "Popular" BN1 Mason Pearson model distributes that user's own sebaceous oil through their hair, presenting a healthy sheen to an otherwise dry, damaged, brittle, deficient in quality texture head of hair. The motive behind brushing dry hair before retiring for sleep at night is logical: it's relaxing, while also giving a rich lubrication, allowing several hours of absorption before most mornings we commonly shampoo and condition during our wake-me-up shower.

With any natural bristle brush, your attention above all must remain focused on the scalp. A mistake people often make: that insufficient tapping approach when brushing, bouncing off the scalp using quick motions.

Another general misunderstanding when brushing: ripping through the hair haphazardly, starting strokes mid-shaft. Instead, begin detangling at your ends, working then upward. Once all snarls and tangles have been removed properly, you're then ready for actual brushing.

Bristles of the brush should continuously stay in contact with your scalp until that firm, even stroke has been completed.

Start at the front, temples and forehead, brushing back toward that neckline nape section, following throughout your hair's length — count fifty strokes, you're halfway done.

In order to brush hair opposite step one, (reversing direction) tip your head forward, nose pointed toward toes; start brushing now from this neckline nape section toward the front temples and forehead area, repeating again another fifty strokes throughout hair's length.

By dragging outward this sebaceous oil onto your hair's shaft and ends, you will additionally exfoliate dry skin at the scalp, creating a healthy follicle, also stimulating blood circulation, producing shinier, thicker hair.

One hundred brush strokes every night — you knew that already though anyhow; that's what grandmothers are for, and accessible Mr. Haute Coiffure, making certain everyone remembers.

✝

✝

Spying About

Although widely seen, I have an isolated incident to comment on, transpiring before a recent business trip at the airport's TSA security screening. Removing my shoes there, I realized Jeanette and LouLou had already walked through the metal detector, passing a woman ahead of me who succeeded filling five bins, flowing over with much she should've checked or left at home. Retrieving my shoes, belt, and satchel, I located the nearest chair right beside a stainless steel TSA security table. I looked down, tied one set of laces, then the other; turning upward, at my left, noticed a uniformed, blue rubber-gloved agent inspecting that woman's possessions who'd been standing before me, detained alongside his examination area. He opened her carry-on luggage, dividing those contents in half for easy layout, publicly exposing this woman's articles.

Had we not arrived so promptly for our domestic flight, two hours early, I wouldn't have lingered, staying seated awhile longer, struck by curiosity. I pretended to reorganize our boarding passes and personal items before putting them back into my satchel; sort of felt like the bungling spy. Couldn't believe what I witnessed, motioning my eyes toward Jeanette's direction, as she might find diversion in getting an eyeful, too.

The first items that grabbed my attention: her round brushes, two of which were about identical in size — super stocky, having heat-conducting metal barrels. I've never used one; however, I am aware many women need them, trying to convince their bane-of-existence textured curls and waves into straight submission, temporarily at least before any summer humidity, autumn fog, winter snow, or spring rain.

The TSA agent wasn't concerned as I was with her round brushes; he left them in their wide elastic bands which stabilized each into place. What baffled me more than her prized round brush collection was a realization that manufacturers had developed specialized luggage based on adequate statistical data implying high maintenance women require uniquely designed wheeling carts for their beauty everything nonsense.

One bottle after another; within seconds various wet hair products stood on the table, around six — scratch that, at least seven — this TSA agent was still pulling bottles out when I got up. He tried to explain her liquid containers each exceeded TSA's allotted three-ounce regulation, requiring they be checked. Reacting vehemently, the woman barked she had already paid for two pieces of stowed luggage, $25 each, which meant she'd require to check that mobile salon or dump her wet stuff. She chose to gather five filthy plastic bins of essential who-cares-what, return through security, head toward her airline's ticket counter, stand in line yet again, pay another $25 — amounting $75 — enjoying TSA and their primordial system once again.

Prior to passing the security scanner, I admired her Burberry rain hat in one of those bins that she'd apparently plopped on top with a matching scarf and coat underneath. As we stood ready for boarding at gate A8, the final image of this dreadfully burdened traveler I recollect was that Burberry hat concealing practically every hair on her head. Did I have empathy for Lady Burberry? Sure did, felt like shaking her shoulders, telling this absolute stranger she needed none of those hair products; nevertheless, can't explain rational reasoning to an addict, no matter how much you try.

Mentioning this was a circumstance set apart, what I gained personal knowledge of seemed like ridiculous decision-making; if only Lady Burberry could have been able to step back from herself watching what I'd seen. When a person is that heavily invested in unattainable perfect appearances, they'll continue carting about costly beauty products, swelling so much, making it impossible to hand-carry this load on their own accord.

Don't know about you, but I've forever had the travel bug. Many state they'd favor sticking close to home — what might we suppose, do they actually favor sticking around their house, or can't honestly fathom how non-complex packing can be?

While boarded at LAX waiting for departure, only ten minutes late, toward SFO, I gazed outside my window, seeing hard evidence of what those opting to remain in town may also have issue with: baggage carriers tossing passenger luggage about as rubbish collectors do. An hour and twenty minutes later at San Francisco International, four of them yukked it up with each other — finding myself instantly irritated, watching one laughing while throwing our bags off the plane's conveyor belt onto SFO's tarmac.

Just for amusement, let's tag this enactment something different — Buffoonery sounds acceptable — dedicated to all who've experienced luggage without defect checking in, discovering elsewhere upon arrival, receiving strollers, what have you, inside the jetway, maybe later at baggage carousel, that we then had one, possibly more, of our wheels broken, handle partially torn off, zipper popped, corners tattered, or smeared from grease. Describing those luggage handlers as buffoons urges a signal — travelers mustn't overpack.

✝

✟

Bon Voyage

When leaving home we'll pack what feels like a temporary representation of our identities; indirectly this does qualify as B-list ranking under the global beauty umbrella, further expressing how less is more. The trick: having one carry-on bag and laptop if your smartphone won't suffice. Most well-known hotels offer executive services including wifi, computers, printer, scanner, and fax machine.

My circumstance traveling is distinctly unavoidable; business trips require I pack cutting shears inside checked luggage, no way around it. Whatever you can do to prevent anyone else beside a blue rubber-gloved TSA agent from rifling through your possessions makes the airport process practically pleasant.

Improvise — why pack another pair of socks and underwear if those you're wearing, rinsed, squeezed, hung dry overnight, possibly finish drying by your room's built-in blow dryer come morning?

How many others besides myself have had issues using travel-size plastic containers, those leaking through faulty

folding nozzles, defective caps unscrewing themselves
while shifting, and bottles occasionally cracking?
Whatever you do, don't skimp by using inferior hotel
shampoo, conditioner, or body lotion. Short on time,
forgetting to purchase those lame travel-size bottles
— instead squirt preferred personal shampoo (small
individual application amounts) into the corner of a clear
plastic baggie, knot tightly just past its capacity, snip off
that bag's remaining excess; secure others for conditioner,
body lotion, and toothpaste; place inside an extra-thick
Ziploc bag while traveling, hermetically sealed once
checked in at your accommodations.

Not every hotel provides complimentary slippers, so
pack lightweight flip-flops; stepping barefoot on public
traffic room carpet, bathroom floors, and shower is
begging for trouble.

A full-on exclusive outfit set aside for your exercise of
choice can be eliminated, don't pack it. Instead request
an extra king-size flat sheet from hotel housekeeping,
have a field day on your unfolded white starched surface,
practicing yoga, or reminisce using traditional junior
high calisthenics. A couple days away from the stationary
bike or treadmill won't end anybody's life. Amazing
how determined convicts can stay ripped, maintaining
twelve-pack shape without ever using elliptical training
machines. An HD flat screen in your room during hotel
workouts surely beats some crummy translucent acrylic
thirteen-inch black-and-white TV set inside a six-by-
eight concrete prison cell.

Select wisely your wardrobe — fabric, color, style, and versatility. If clothing choices are difficult on a daily basis at home, it won't be any less stressful packing, high chances even more so.

✝

BY JEHR SCHIAVO
WRITING AS GERARD SAINT D'ANGELO

✝

40K FLUSHED AWAY

Yesterday I was reminded why, in a big way, someone should disclose how inferior an enormous cross-section of women sense themselves. The ensuing material found Mr. Haute Coiffure much difficulty digesting.

There wasn't any doubt the client I'm about to speak of would be eccentric; she'd postponed her first appointment two weeks ago en route, thirty minutes late; Jeanette rescheduled another visit. Eventually I greeted this woman inside our building's lobby waiting area; she was standing in front of the floor-to-ceiling glass window at ground level, her hair visibly a Grace Coddington frizzy silhouette against that bright daylight's backdrop. During the next ninety minutes together I obtained understanding that she was angelic, in stark contrast to this witch's mane my scissors would address.

After taking her black blazer, I glanced briefly at the label while hanging it and saw a partial 'Cartney — each button blended, nearly evaporating into this garment, rounded yet petite, tastefully covered by matching fabric.

She had the resources to afford a key article of clothing, utopian as you'll find — brunches or funerals and everything between; more importantly an eye-choosing Stella McCartney, who continues proving herself. Sir Paul may've pulled influential strings, but his daughter ain't messing around.

Hands are the giveaway; age can remain ambiguous guessing by facial features, although usually determined after a gentle handshake during introduction with my notice of both. She might have been older, yet I'm gracious; I'll settle the difference by saying our ages are within a few years of each other. Rarely a woman over fifty pulls off what looks appropriate, aesthetically so, wearing hair several inches past her shoulders. When breast size requires offsetting (obvious example, Dolly Parton), longer hair camouflages gazungas. My client sported neither implants nor blonde wig, unless she hid them at home, out of sight.

Her harsh chemically-induced monochromatic jet black hair, I came to understand, was covering what she described as turning white prematurely upon thirty; scheduling the colorist every three weeks, spending approximately $100 per visit — news flash — thievery, people! If you give a small child an apron, spatula, and mixing bowl filled with icing, they will easily frost cupcakes 'til their little fingers cramp; so could anyone applying hair color, my client no exception. For approximately $15 she'd be better off stopping into her nearest beauty supply, asking the sales assistant to locate one pair of rubber gloves, an applicator bottle, a two-ounce tube containing Morticia black tint, and developer. Why pay one hundred bucks for somebody else to destroy your hair when you can pocket $85 — less gratuity, parking, gas and aggravation — by injuring it less yourself.

As for flattery, the subtle approach prevails. Why ever inform any person their hair looks and feels similar to a witch's broom; we may not have the slightest clue how closely associated that shoddy colorist might be. I'll avoid accusing anyone of having ruined anything, even if they have.

Forty-five minutes into our initial appointment she mentioned her enjoyment seeing beautiful women in fashion magazines. Upon further investigation, told me she admired Gisele Bündchen — more accurately, desired Gisele's personal beauty. I responded, pointing out most fashion models, other than an exclusive handful, are mere kids, late teens into their, at tops, early twenties. What shall fifty-year and older women do aside from splurging on a Stella McCartney blazer to feel younger, that which actually doesn't harm them — hair thrashed by excessive heat and chemical services, or furthermore negative side effects receiving injectable fillers?

Aging elegantly according to French designer Jean Paul Gaultier was unveiled during Paris fashion week: his 2014/2015 Autumn/Winter ready-to-wear collection, featuring female and male runway models

rocking grey mohawks, silver bouffants, while also
nudging boundaries redefining beauty, playing up white
flowing tresses.

✝

BY JEHR SCHIAVO
WRITING AS GERARD SAINT D'ANGELO

✝

M.O.

This, if I do say so myself, seems a golden moment to make an informal introduction of the Jehrcut. It's what others would classify as a haircut — mine is, however isn't. Should I in an uncompromising situation find dispute, interrogated when the Jehrcut originated, that answer couldn't be determined by any one such specific date. Who brought forth the term is patent. If I were that intellectual hired by Webster's defining whatever previously unheard-of word, there would not be an excess of more than several words forming a concise definition.

Why clients are asked by the stylist how long or short they desire their hair dates back thousands of moons ago — this ludicrous and antiquated approach has been my long-standing observation's quandary. Tip of the iceberg, set off my avalanche, erupting a tidal wave's creative process; now, nearly five hundred moons, hundreds stir substantial credibility, I've again estimated an even figure — "four hundred and eighty moon phases" doesn't quite resonate, does it?

Where can a client go for professional advice regarding their hair? The answer, I once thought, was that salon of high regard. Whether remaining lackadaisical or mediocre through inexperience, most stylists inquire, their client directs them, that particular appointment is then complete, with the recipient of a hairstyle resembling photographs from magazines they'd shown, if not tried describing. Stay home, cut it yourself, either way this isn't any greater extent different than hair snipped at demanded lengths; a simplistic haircut — you cutting, or those stylists asking what they should do.

No one refers to time lapsed by moon cycles these days; I'll join the masses, too. In 1977, one subtle lesson made a lasting impression on me, discovering myself closely viewing my assigned stylist's client's footwear during her consultation, which I was privy to as an apprentice. A person's inherent style could often be detected by the shoes they select. Most clients prepare in advance what they will wear for the initial consultation and subsequent service. I wouldn't say dressed wearing their Sunday best — ideally, that meaningful persona we as experts can then embellish.

Half that initial lesson at this moment appears obsolete, with the advent of compulsory smart devices featuring digital clocks, yet there is merit in commenting on a person's wristwatch, smartwatches included. Jewelry changes, for many every day, but the wrist timepiece usually doesn't.

While a client remains clothed in their salon-issued
robe, drape, or both, not much personal style is exposed.
Grandiloquent salons employ uniformed assistants
who escort clients to their stylists already robed. Today
I've the luxury of considering my patron's total style
upon initial greeting; they're dressed head-to-toe.
Mine is as notable an unsalon I couldn't ever have
imagined dreaming of — a pop-up atelier with routine
designations in Los Angeles, San Francisco, and New
York, honoring special locations upon request. For those
elsewhere, not visiting Mr. Haute Coiffure, probability
states your cell phone clock is adequate, replacing that
once-indispensable wristwatch, leaving but only a single
pair of shoes, illustrating tellingly to the stylist what
fashion sense you possess.

It could be you rest within that majority of clients, a
head protruding from the stylist's cutting cape. Next this
stylist inquires, "What would you like to do?" — odds are
not in your favor. If the style doesn't come across quite
right (could have performed better on hair with different
texture, possibly framing another face, maybe you don't
dress that hip; even more painful, this cut's too severe or
conservative) that's a result of any haircut, not someone
else's Jehrcut.

✝

✝

Intermezzo

Many reading at this stage could be thinking various thoughts to themselves.

"When's he gonna shut up about how rotten everybody's hair is?"

"Yes, I'd love to know what Mr. Haute Coiffure suggests changing, if we are supposing true his spunky conversation."

"Absolutely my thought, okay, our hair is in horrible disrepair, I can see for myself it's not cut well."

"We can't ever style it in that way the stylist had us looking before leaving their salon, now what, Mr. Haute Coiffure?"

Every comment is an improvement; before opening any page here, you've, I believe, had these parallel thoughts, but some percent, for reasons unknown, continue to style hair the way you have: in that identical manner since borrowing Mom's products, round brushes, blow dryer, and irons from age twelve.

If you're starting to become impatient, which I'll take

as a compliment, I commend you. That craving for solid answers has made your appetite ravenous; you'd on the contrary be more partial to hear straightforward solutions.

Most of those prior lines were speculation on my part; wouldn't I be a marvel, having the ability to foresee thoughts, past, present, and future — no one will, because nobody can. Psychics, clairvoyants, soothsayers, what have you, they'll also steal if we permit them — preying without remorse on those susceptible, another loosely linked offshoot in this beauty industry's environment of hocus pocus sorcery.

Whoever concedes at this juncture that I've triggered awareness regarding negative aspects causing perpetual dilemma beyond poor quality hair, bravissimo. For others these valuable findings may someday eventually resonate; let's hope everyone gets caught up with each other — this however isn't a foot race. Matter of fact, if you haven't already, flip through this book, front to back cover — no pictures, illustrations, or diagrams, bullet points, graphs, nor numbered procedures — strange? Actually not. What would anyone expect as an example, a photograph of Catherine Deneuve in her prime?

Hair is an extension of ourselves. Much of how I've gained life knowledge wasn't information given — undoubtedly, some was. It has been what I acquired through experience, those are the lessons I'll solemnly wish not ever to forget. Therefore, read between these lines; I may periodically tap you on the shoulder with a few tidbits as alternative options, while primarily thinking for yourself. Permit Mr. Haute Coiffure, the utmost outsider, an inside purview into this bohemian direction, style's ease and sustainability, arriving through that momentum of surprise without pictures, illustrations, or diagrams, bullet points, graphs, nor numbered procedures.

Millions could say I've neglected differentiating between women and men, the general sense about ourselves exhibited by appearances.

"He's barely said two words about men, what does he think, they're above his rebellious criteria?"

Mr. Haute Coiffure is neither sexist nor biased; accruing as many buildings with "Trump" in gilded bold letters glaring across its facade doesn't make this billionaire exempt from bad taste concerning his personal looks. Johnny Depp, God love him, may be among Hollywood's wealthiest men, although this didn't afford him profound style either, unless his gypsy apparel seems convincing. No sane person would argue overhearing this comment, "They're icons; each should spend his money exactly how he pleases." That I won't disagree with, though a lacquered 70s used car salesman comb-over hairdo, wearing white under eye highlighter, and bronzer devalue Donald Trump's bespoke suits, seemingly bought on discount for seventy-nine bucks at Jos. A. Bank. Depp's adolescent infatuation with Keith Richards — who hadn't ever displayed any shame, a septuagenarian wearing eyeliner, even if he cofounded the Rolling Stones — should've at no time inspired Johnny's eyelining treatment, whether tattooed permanently or cosmetically, mimicking Keith. Paul Newman, dapper guy, fared extremely well. Sundance, on the other hand, ain't a Kid no more. Why foxy Robert Redford felt the uncontrollable determination to have an eye lift is mind-boggling beyond my imagination. I'm almost positive his vain decision won't ever be a topic of discussion during any film festival opening parties coming soon to an independent theater near you. Billy Crystal, what had he envisioned, wasn't the mass acclaim for comic genius enough to bolster his deflated ego, preventing a full-blown face lift?

Thus we witness Bruce Jenner, a cultural crossover — beauty for sale, going once, twice, sold to Caitlyn, affording the best doctors money could buy. Can anybody make sense by what striking face we saw watching The Pope of Greenwich Village turned into, seeing Mickey Rourke presently? Nope, you're thoroughly error-free, aging naturally has become practically evil; it's arrantly acceptable for men to distort themselves grotesquely as well; supreme talent portrayed on the exterior doesn't necessarily mean they're completely healthy inside.

✝

✝

Pimps and Whores

Who doesn't sense sheer excitement when a much-awaited film at long last gets released? We'll dash in the car, driving off to enjoy this fantastic movie. Could be other interests — music, dance, theater — which stimulate passion; somebody, a group you've always loved, is scheduled soon, everybody's going. Our instinct hankers after entertainment.

Before anyone pours out the passenger door speeding around this next curve, as your driver I should forewarn everyone: hang on, buckle up, we're moving into certified analogy jurisdiction. There was a period when I spoke using only analogies if I'd determined well-reasoned inference, explaining myself otherwise seemed impossible. Two drawbacks were apparent: that frequency developed into an uncontrollable habit; second, most significantly, I wound up actually confusing who this was I'd been desperately trying to communicate with. I weaned myself toward incrementally fewer doses until the present moment, restraining nothing more than a minute longer, taking presently this opportunity for any indulgences befitting. No need to fret, I have a lead right foot, but my left one is consistently above the brake, everybody's safe, could be herky-jerky ahead, yet nobody should require traction being hospitalized.

All thirsty vehicles covering the earth's surface necessitate gasoline, converted from crude oil through ominous refineries. Popular faces, secured through advertising endorsement contracts, represent each make and model — an eco-unfriendly alignment between the unsustainable beauty industry and voracious fuel energy consumption; we insist upon buying crackbrained, often detrimental matter we're insidiously sold. As an example, Justin Bieber and Katy Perry appear on extended television commercials, promoting benzoyl peroxide and salicylic acid — Proactiv's main pernicious ingredients.

Has humanity's denial level become filled to the brim? The establishment refuses to accept accountability, observing resources are becoming diminished in oil fields and under offshore platforms. Mankind has stood by several decades waging tragic wars over it. Our inherent selfish reasoning continues spoiling this planet — as do multimillionaire celebrities prostituting themselves, feeding the public their next endorsement.

Detroit, once an iconic American force to be reckoned with, crippled; Gulf Coast cities aroused pity, barely standing after Katrina, followed by the British Petroleum pummeling; skies above Mumbai, Beijing, and Phoenix cast a malignant shade. Those free from

hypocrisy take responsible measures — walk, skate, ride
bikes, and use public transportation. Celebrities should
display probity enhancing life, opposed to Matthew
McConaughey, yet another whore endorsing Lincoln's
MKX gas guzzler. Many understand deep down, it's an
epic battle, immensely greater by proportion than David
and Goliath. We still persevere knowing this courageous
changing of the old guard can occur, however tedious
a process. Sooner than you'd guess, better-improved
vehicles relying completely on renewable energy will
replace what delivered previous harmful effects to
humans and our mothership. Good riddance, crude
oil; barrels worth top dollar currently see their prices
plummeting. Clean power made available by creative
minds — Elon Musk, the new heavyweight world
champion innovator. A historic haul, from rationing gas
nearly forty years ago to bitter tragedy, those soldiers
severely maimed alongside their brothers' fatalities —
immeasurable family suffering, over coveted oil.

KISS hasn't ever held any interest for me whatsoever
— schlock rock on their best day, obnoxious as they're
made. A fortune built pontificating the quantity
of fornication; his elongated tongue dripping stage
blood evolved into Gene Simmons reality TV series
glorifying plastic surgery, yet another deplorable period
in television entertainment. A barbaric vehicle laying in
wait with bated breath, Simmons tapped into the beauty
industry's insatiable quest, refueling A&E's empty tank.

Hollywood's advertising temptation, its demise in

code of values, occurred right before our fascinated eyes. Yesteryear's mega superstars slowly but surely began disappearing; neither Jack Nicholson nor Meryl Streep peddle products, unlike George "Lake Como" Clooney selling Italians an array, dairy to cologne. Rapacity, the nasty commodity — hot one though: thirty million per picture demanded by Academy Award-preferred stars. Big splashy opening weekend box office sales dipped, streaming directly onto our devices, while independent film and animation grows more successful than Hollywood ever anticipated.

Major beauty corporations lost interest hiring fashion models. The cash-hungry monster opted for substitution, using their advertising vehicle's weapon of mass consumption, any celebrity near or far: pop, opera, rock, country, athlete, stage, television, and silver screen.

America's resplendent entertainment industry's reputation nosedived, compliments of the beauty industry. Burt Reynolds was paid to act. His hideous appearance on-screen following a face-lift prompted Joe Schmo also to have plastic surgery. Is it not the entertainer's role to amuse us? Just because their agent suggests they present themselves younger, that doesn't imply my client should dye her hair black, attempting the likeness of Dita Von Teese, Demi Moore, or Cher's wigs.

As a professional on movie sets, fashion, photo, or music video shoots, and runway shows, I discovered myself amid an assortment of specialists connected capturing this image the public swoons over. The personnel invariably comprises more than one hairstylist, makeup artists, scads for wardrobe, lighting designers, photographer or cinematographer plus their team, art directors, concluded with computer image enhancement — voilà, Sarah Jessica Parker's immediate reversal, thirty from fifty.

It's cruel that society should spurn themselves in such a manner, believing they will walk into any beauty salon, hand the stylist magazines, indicating whatever entertainer consumers want to resemble. Many's acceptance of how they look through aging had not proved effective; stepping outdoors, googling plastic surgeon possibilities, this future patient then begs for a nose similar to Jennifer Lawrence, pouty Naomi Campbell lips, ninnies matching Scarlett Johansson's voluptuous rack this year, sometime thereafter requesting her reduction — peach-sized Charlize Theron cup.

By this sarcastic interjection, most probably are aware, aging doesn't sit well with entertainers; relatively speaking, mainstream cosmetic surgery doesn't date back all that many years. Maintaining youthful beauty is a pressure cooker's ultimate exhaustion; Norma Jean's candle in the wind blew out; Miley, Selena, Paris, Britney, Kylie continued pushing their envelope; Heath, who knows, no turning back there. Meanwhile, our clocks keep ticking, while many celebrities pay through the teeth hoping to go counterclockwise. Lawless, those responsible with platform run amok, projecting unrealistic body and face standards. The Federal Trade Commission can't crack down because Congress hasn't legislated their proposed Truth in Advertising Act. An executive, enabling boosterism for Julia Roberts' next box office hit, orders his creative director to airbrush her neck beneath the chin area a smidgen more. *Eat, Pray, Love* me the way I am.

Whoever differs in opinion is entitled, absolutely, your privilege without question. But, if this is yours, defending actions Mr. Haute Coiffure detects censurable, understand that I have visible beliefs, guided divinely as a beautician adventurer should.

Mine, vouching on behalf of me, didn't always travel with my alter ego Mr. Haute Coiffure. We in time respectfully gathered rapport with each other when I conducted business affairs managing my career alone before Jeanette's miraculous arrival. Without doubt there will be plenty quick to judge, having firm convictions that I and Mr. Haute Coiffure are naysayers, carrying outlandish, paranoid beliefs bordering conspiracy theories. Those sensing dubious merit, to you, factual submission: Hollywood's film and television entertainment industry facilitates an elaborate advertising campaign for the annual quarter-trillion-dollar beauty conglomeration.

✝

+

NY, NY 10065

Between 1991 and 2001, I conducted business making
Manhattan house calls, having a permanent studio
cutting clients in San Francisco, with an alternative
space for my Los Angeles patrons. New York City was
where this particular story took place, that's the location.
Occasionally I'll present myself at a client's home or
place of business, be it office, restaurant, bar, backstage,
boutique, hotel suite, and whatnot. No other modus
operandi within my trade will set any stylist on an efficient
course toward succumbing to a client by walking inside,
specifically their personal dwelling. You'll know within
minutes, after having not ever before been invited into
someone's home, those extraordinary details you wouldn't
in a lifetime previously have surmised about them.

Certain Upper East Side tree-lined Manhattan blocks
remain standouts, exceptional buildings I've visited —
64th between Park and Madison is one of many. I found
myself returning Uptown, cutting two quite dissimilar
clients at their apartments' different plush addresses

on the very same street. As any freelance hairstylist
could suppose, receiving that message requesting an
appointment for a high-rank employee of L'Oréal isn't the
everyday occurrence; discovering she's North America's
Public Relations Director at Giorgio Armani Fragrance —
rarely if ever do such opportunities come knocking.

Wasn't pleasant, my client's demeanor across the
street closer to Madison Avenue — married old money;
husband bought their over-decorated three-bedroom,
formal dining room, library, and maid's quarters, a
resplendent residence by most New York City standards,
while my vivacious PR client lived seemingly carefree,
renting her comfy, cluttered apartment; both women
were exact representations of those distinct abodes.

The married client was of those quintessential
melodramatic Upper East Side women — for what it's
worth, hadn't ever hoisted a single finger. Placing myself
inside that fussy home was difficult to deal with. Our
personalities clashed as if dropping a lit match on dry
scrub brush; I ignited an inferno she'd found detestable
— nonetheless, she kept scheduling appointments.
Further east down the street, Vivacious and Comfy,
within those seconds getting inside, closing her door,
triple-locking deadbolts behind me, I felt completely
welcome at once — exactly how she'd grown accustomed
to treating others representing L'Oréal products.

Some folks can't stomach their work; a smaller
percentage won't have enough hours in any given day
doing what they adore. This Public Relations Director

split straight down the center; I couldn't figure out if she loathed her demanding, no-real-time-for-life position or relished it, virtually muddled, consequently that apartment's strewn epitome.

✝

BY JEHR SCHIAVO
WRITING AS GERARD SAINT D'ANGELO

✝

TEN BILLION-DOLLAR ITALIAN MAN

Eensy teensy weensy years forming decades, fashion
designer labels began creeping into Hollywood's
opulent budgets. Hadn't been that way watching
Gone with the Wind, not a visible label there; however,
by 1980's *American Gigolo*, Richard Gere modeled
blatantly, swaggering Giorgio Armani menswear before
our movie ticket eyes. Close shots of his wardrobe,
fastidiously laid out, revealed labels whose name had
also then scrolled up during credits.

Don't anyone dare address Giorgio Armani, Giorgio.
Make no mistake, subordinates must always receive
him as "Mister Armani." Such a preposterous degree of
propriety was partial impetus giving Mr. Haute Coiffure's
sardonic title — alongside ancient clients' addressing
renowned male hairstylists prior to Sassoon. Mr. Bubbles,
Mr. Coffee and Mr. Clean might too take their bows.
Even former heads of state don't warrant this strict
decorum, as egotistically maniacal, highfalutin' designers
often define themselves. Young Giorgio Americanized

83

his titlement; I wonder if he obviously understood "Signore Armani" wasn't going to cut it in the United States, that same way his standard Italian garments did.

Should skeptics gripe, "He's such a liar; Giorgio Armani's clothes are to the hilt gorgeous."

Tour major Italian cities, Turin to Palermo; you'll discover quality hand-tailoring that transcends Armani's factory-made products. Artisans' affection, steeped by centuries, passed through generations, total respect and enthusiasm of craft — unlike Giorgio's relentless pursuit in branding, yet another blasé Macy's home collection. The man's stricken with entrepreneurial fever; I'll have to assume consumers don't already own enough greige.

Spray your common everyday household insecticide on a piece of paper; do the blind test, spraying another swatch with Armani men's cologne — allow each to dry, then sniff. (I'm not participating in that challenge.) My Vivacious and Comfy PR client loaded me up with a ton of Giorgio Armani beauty products for men; she had enough stashed in her apartment to drown George Hamilton. How disgusting can any man smell that he require an arsenal of products, those I later found after opening equally abhorrent as bug repellant.

Manufacturers bottling Armani fragrance apparently fill hoards of other companies' orders as well, using then that customer's glitterati-branded packaging. Those revolting perfume odors cause me migraine headaches at lightning speed, essential oil included, especially patchouli; breathing anywhere within that stink's vicinity

leaves a poisonous flavor on my tongue and throat.
Strolling past houses of ill repute within Paris' Pigalle,
having overtones blending liquor and spew, would smell
agreeable in comparison.

Beauty is in the eye of a cameraman's lens. Film
directors spend crazed hours, to the Earth's end,
capturing an impressive Baccarat crystal chandelier
hovering above a winding Calacatta marble staircase —
his stunning leading actress' flowing decent preserved,
wearing reminiscent couture gown, your selection,
unequivocal black Balenciaga, classic white Dior,
exceptional gold Valentino. We remember that year's
lavish motion picture scenes, well-positioned for Oscar's
much-awaited evening, having our votes ready, best
wardrobe included. Red carpet pre-ceremonies drag on
for the duration it takes to present that year's Academy
Awards, a two-hour feature-length fashion designer
advertising maneuver — Hollywood's successful and
profitable marriage with Madison Avenue.

Has this cherished gala gone completely bonkers?
If so, are not the masses obliged to speak out, voicing
powers of argument? Perhaps in a not-so-distant year
the Academy of Motion Picture Arts and Sciences will
enforce restrictions which prohibit pandering, as their
annual event continues to devolve, surpassing vulgar
levels; should Anna Wintour be seated front row, seating
Cate Blanchett behind four, five, even six rows back?

Returning to the New York story: this drizzly night
I found myself cabbing again toward 64th Street from

26th at Waterside Plaza — partially drenched clothing, my gust-swept umbrella inside-out, satchel, cutting cape, comb and scissors. Vivacious and Comfy buzzed me in; I rode the polished antique elevator car up, hearing another floor away her voice intermixed with young women giggling, having a blast. What can happen when entering a client's home, as everybody other than myself consumed alcohol, doesn't typically occur cutting clients in the salon, nor do adding two of her girlfriends who weren't leaving. They were joining Vivacious and Comfy at Radio City Music Hall afterward for the Academy Awards simulcast party — Giorgio Armani, best fragrance in a film.

Roll credits; bear witness for yourself the dominance of absurdity, a scent's artificial presence on screen. Promoting what is invisible, Giorgio, your dexterous marketing campaign was ingenious. Congratulations, now go ahead, toodle-oo, buy yourself an upgraded luxury superyacht; however, you ought to consider developing another Mediterranean sunscreen; your abbronzatura has been a tad on the leathery side.

✝

☩

Razzmatazz

Now and again the unusually warm-hearted intellectual
patron arrives; from whom inner beauty magically
radiates, sending my scissors into heaven's glory,
unobstructed bliss. Were these shears yours, not ever
taught technically how hair should get cut, it would
surprise her more than yourself that she could appear
just as lovely when you, the novice, are done cutting.

Aside from complimenting her, which effectually
gathered minor convincing on my part at our first
consultation, the following line could also benefit
as additional explanation: A nectarine seldom lands
far from its wooden trunk, unless this odd long-ago
ovule blew uphill, growing there, bearing fruit later
tumbling downhill.

Few and far between as a nectarine tree planted firmly
upon hilltop will I be called for by the interested patron
two thousand miles away. Factor in one round-trip ticket
from Chicago destination west, a Christmas holiday
nestled inside the Berkeley Hills amidst her warm-hearted

intellectual daughter and prized assembled family, soon
creating elements of *On Golden Pond* strain, adding too
another test, her mother's Jehrcut.

Hey there, hold your Clydesdales, before everyone goes
galloping through forestland by open sleigh for a holiday
Jehrcut, follow here these details as they unfold; you'll
within those twinkles of upcoming insight understand that
complications can be — like this situation regarding my
new Midwestern client, nearly ninety years in the making.

Between extreme bluster and subzero temperatures,
honestly, there isn't much I'd guarantee a personal
recommendation visiting Chicago during its frigid
winter. I worked there, attending America's Beauty
Show convention for three days late-January many
years ago; didn't leave the hosting hotel once. Afterward
I left O'Hare on a flight bound toward JFK with
uncontrollable shivers, accompanied by aches with
fever of one hundred and two. Plenty of people who
know report the North Shore is one Chicago enclave
characterized by prestigious real estate — where Mother
in Windy City originated, centering her life there,
forever and a day.

I hadn't ever before met Mother, though gathered she
was well-to-do, resilient, but petrified by change. Warm-
hearted Intellectual Daughter relayed that Mother
and her long-standing friends shared many delightful
anecdotes, quite often calling one another "darling."
Mother, I was told, wore Princess Leia braided semi-
spherical mounds at each side of the head; unpinned,

taking them down and combed through, Mother's hair reached her tailbone. I'd been also aware, underneath her chemical over-processing Mother had white hair, which she insisted on tinting a reddish color — could be auburn, maybe strawberry, doesn't matter. Hers penalized, chemically treated, that condition's quality undoubtedly punished by whatever shade dye had been applied. Considering this exceptional length and significant lifetime paid to have it processed, I knew her hair had been severely tortured in Chicago.

When a prisoner of war finds release, they don't automatically run into their family's loving extended arms; there's that certain interval they're cared for, physically examined, mentally observed, ensuring reunification will rest harmoniously, returning then alongside everyone at home. If Mother musters up true meaning to free herself — refusing imprisonment's bondage of her own hair — such a sacrifice would be an impressive, monumental feat.

Dramatically altering the hairstyle of an elderly person is a privilege which shouldn't be taken lightly. Here on, I've made my decision for Mr. Haute Coiffure, I'm cutting much of Mother's hair off. Warm-hearted Intellectual Daughter I hope has a camera including video capability; for all one knows we'll cast this Jehrcut on YouTube, transforming grandmotherly Princess Leia into twenty-first century sophisticate.

Elsewhere on Chicago's South Side, some ninety-odd years ago, automobile horns emitted the sound of a

tender goose's rough handling; flappers affected knee-
length tassel dresses, adorned by extra-lengthy single-
strand pearls, and meticulously placed roaring twenties
finger-waved hair — precise setting where famished men
obeyed Al Capone.

Not very long thereafter, Mother — way back then,
Precocious North Shore Schoolgirl — played with
porcelain toy figurines, appeared for dinner when called;
no one dressed casually, not even she — buckle-accented
leather shoes, crinoline petticoat, jumper frock over crisp
long-sleeve blouse, having both frills and lace, ample
velvet bow securing hair from her alabaster face.

On occasion Precocious North Shore Schoolgirl's
mother and father darted out after dinner, though
not before tucking her in. Both parents instructed her
nanny before leaving — painting then, in formal wear,
Chicago Town vividness it pined for following America's
Great Depression. They reveled hearing lively Count
Basie, Duke Ellington; later into predawn dancing
slowed, being serenaded, "ladies and gentlemen, the
incomparable Ella Fitzgerald."

She grew statuesque through the years; her hair
too had grown, sitting upon it during class attending
Chicago's outstanding private schools; by senior year
Miss North Shore Schoolgirl was voted student body
president. She fell head-over-heels in love her first year
at a neighboring university — unusually gifted with
whatever he touched: their team's pigskin football,
treating patients while doing rounds between wrapping

up his taxing dissertation, or bracing our young woman's swooning fall.

Euphoric midas lad altogether delighted by his radiant "I do," now Mrs. North Shore — decked out on their wedding day: unending Mulberry silk, Duchess satin, and Chantilly lace trim; her bridal gown enveloped each photographic frame. Standing before altar, God, and man at Holy Name Cathedral, midas lad peered, raising his bride's headdress veil. This incepted hairstyle marked her non-ceasing identical pair of braided semi-spherical mounds. Positively wouldn't part with them; she couldn't wear that invaluable wedding dress daily throughout life, choosing instead her storybook specially designed hairstyle. Perhaps this nuptial hairdo had been an awe-inspiring event's styling answer — the affluent bride's dreaded question posed before her hired hairdresser, his client's pre-wedding nerves jangled; be that as it may, triumphed he did.

Dr. and Mrs. North Shore proudly cohabitated, rearing children who thrived, also attending their parents' same private blue-chip Chicago schools, earning prominent degrees, marrying equally well, prospering further, blessing them with healthy grandkids.

Such bitter surprise a short time ago, ninety-four-year-old midas grandfather, Dr. North Shore, suffers after his debilitating stroke. Mrs. North Shore had become frail herself, unable to assist her husband. He, now permanently disabled, requires twenty-four-hour care, dependent solely on others. She visits him, however, only a few days every week, this loving wife's rationale nothing of the circumstance her beloved husband hadn't been achingly missed — assuredly he was. Each occasion, stoic Mrs. North Shore gently kisses Dr. North Shore goodbye, after and only then to sob following their visits, wiping those far-too-familiar tears away; once in a blue moon he'll remember his adoring wife of sixty-nine bliss-filled years.

She'll stay close, within an arm's reach of Dr. North Shore in his austere room. Warmer afternoons she'll cover with tartan plaid blanket her husband's icy legs; wheeling him outside under an oak tree, fully grown, she, almost mesmerized, somehow senses each other feeling spry again. Seated on the nursing home bench, holding tenderly husband's pale translucent hand — he, propped upright, just about motionless, paralyzed within his wheelchair — Mrs. North Shore herself during these silent days finds it impossible to envision their days ahead.

Last summer under their tree's fountain of youth, she softly placed his cool fingers on her kind cheek — touching a wife's powerful desire to have life return, by any means at all. His hand lifted sluggishly in manner, inching higher, eventually reaching, cupping her braided semi-spherical mounds. Staring upward into that fabled tree's branches — no, not at her — faintly smiles he does, drawing one river stream, next another, both eyes weeping, speechlessly conveying a disabled husband's sorrow over their stricken, drawn-out year spent apart. For it was on this indelible anniversary date seventy

years prior both said "I do"; each continues reverence in
matrimonial vows, as those sacred seconds exchanging
wedding bands inside Holy Name Cathedral.

His sparse hair replaced by scattered dark freckles
above, hers barely grows — Mrs. North Shore, my client's
mother, currently expecting traumatic cutting.

✝

✦

Stuck in Time

Funny, a woman's strong will, her determination clinging
to that certain pivotal hairstyle, varying in countless
numbers, nearly every female over forty, much more
women than men — him hardly ever, although there
are those one-off instances absolutely. This difference
between the sexes has an explanation you don't really
need my help bringing to your attention: most males wish
they could hang on forever wearing a particular style, yet
balding makes that impossible.

Diehard military types are an excellent example of
how a rough-and-tumble dude who's going bald sticks
with his treasured guns, wearing that crew cut flat-top
even though there's at most peach fur still left up above.
Long as he sees his barber every other week, buzzing two
sharp corner edges forming an illusory flat surface on top,
he's good to go.

Women don't experience alopecia to the extent men
can. When female thinning may often occur later in
their golden years, shaving what's scarcely there isn't her

solution, unless she's a new-modern, observing Vivienne Westwood's choice. Yul Brynner, Telly Savalas, Michael Jordan, and Bruce Willis gave balding acceptance for other men such as myself, another card-carrying member of the international cue ball club.

There in her life was a window of beauty she felt prettiest, appearing happiest; no matter what, until this woman's dying day will do whatever engaging or spending to maintain that former symbol, fully embodying one thousand percent satisfaction seeing herself. Who knows what span this was; in the whopping majority of women it lasts more than one single summer day wearing flowing bridal gown, marrying their own midas lad — for Mrs. North Shore, hers a delicate age at that time, barely finishing her teenage years. The recent arrival whose head pops out her hairstylist's protective drape hardly scratches this woman's exceptional story; why she's so invested with that hairstyle which very well might've been appropriate sometime, somewhere — though woefully, between us, hasn't served as an attractive appearance since Mrs. North Shore's wedding day.

✝

✝

ART AND DIPLOMACY

I've made belittling remarks concerning hairstylists —
how we, myself many years ago included, would bicker
among each other and behind one another's backs.
Same salon, two stylists spitting harsh criticism about a
third individual not present, who's away working on his
or her client; this person then enters their staff room,
whereupon both backstabbers spin, spoon-feeding the
busy stylist strawberries with cream.

Quality, superior in nature, sets up the stage by
degrees and levels professionals find commitment to
— simplified, we will more commonly refer this act as
"possessing integrity." Possibly a situation or two, rather
be realistic saying several times, I have been guilty of
insensitivity. Learned by lopping off those new clients'
waist-length ponytails, thereafter putting their hair
inside Ziploc bags, hadn't however replaced by fair
exchange the true loss. Had Mr. Haute Coiffure not
asked those patrons before cutting two feet of hair if
she'd prefer saving it as a memento, I would've spent that

following hour rotating around my styling chair stepping all over her personal recollections, mere clippings below. During a particularly embarrassing *artiste* period — translation, conceited phase — I wrote in black Sharpie across clear Ziploc bags, containing carefully chosen pieces from that client's shorn hair, identified the date, numbered it 1/1, included my signature, as if this added value to their fee — commissioned works of art.

Somehow I believe Mrs. North Shore and husband deserve much more attention. Craft, remaining exceptionally skillful, is only a portion, so how then does the stylist derive his or her valuation? When this novelty ultimately wore off, signing client's artistic souvenirs — her lifetime investment, case in point, growing Lady Godiva hair — holding fast to what's hers, at last I wholly understood from experience: satisfying the client came through recognizing what she's emotionally prepared for, having bigger importance than my art piece, worn or archival clippings.

There is a balance for Mrs. North Shore and husband; they shall both as it happens reap separate benefits. Mr. Haute Coiffure has vaulted as safekeeping two distinguished gifts, one for each spouse. Mr. Haute Coiffure and I wish you'll take part in, while stumbling on amusement attempting within the privacy of your home.

✝

✝

Start Your Engines

You can purchase haircutting scissors at your local beauty supply, but they won't be Samurai-caliber Japanese shears like those I own — thank goodness, you'd lose a finger — nevertheless yours will get the job done. Combs are necessary, not bulky or having teeth too fine, normal size; ask for an average haircutting comb. Let's round out your fifty bucks: when you're in there pick up a nylon cutting cape; don't mistakenly buy those made of plastic for chemical work, unless whoever's the willing participant doesn't mind sweating to death under that stifling fabric during this haircut experiment.

Apprehensive, eh? No worries, it isn't you who's having a haircut; should anybody be, it's that experimental subject you've convinced to sit in your kitchen, who I add has first right of refusal if either elects the jitters. I'm telling you their hair may, if paying utmost attention isn't your strong suit, necessitate this collaborator's temporary use of hats. A major warning here: profuse bleeding can occur, not injuring the hand stabilizing this sharp instrument you've obtained, but to your other one, securing hair once those precarious scissors begin cutting.

Didn't have any clue a how-to guide was on its way, did you? Unexpectedly shipped in from paradise, that's partly my reasoning to exclude illustrations — it's the wonderful element of surprise, this portion, Look Ma Both Hands. Don't worry, switching this comb from that hand also holding your scissors back into the fingers which seconds ago secured hair while cutting feels clumsy starting out, but by about haircut number fifteen shifting should become much more adaptable.

Practicing on children is a terrible idea. You'll need someone who can sit still; you and your intact fingers will be forever grateful. Try asking an elderly person — they usually have wide-open schedules, welcome sedentary activity, nor mind saving money while living on fixed incomes.

Mrs. North Shore is a generous spender; I've got dibs on her, you'll have to acquire your own paying patron. What are the odds of anybody coming across tailbone-length hair, when braided reaches this person's lower back — from evaluating clients' heads, oodles full, slim to none, you'll be ultra-hard pressed finding your subject.

For nearly ten years Mrs. North Shore had been making frequent complaints to her Warm-hearted Intellectual Daughter about what a difficult ordeal this was, caring for that wealth of hair. Brushing as she always had by evening's end now caused neck problems.

A weekly shampoo using apple cider vinegar wasn't ever easy to begin with; going way-back-when, as her mother washed it in the identical manner eighty-some years earlier. Getting silvery-white roots retouched red every month hadn't been a whole bunch of fun, never was. Another challenge of mine besides Mrs. North Shore's mental stability — what about her sweet husband? Cutting off those Princess Leia head warmers could give Dr. North Shore a coronary thrombosis, and if that didn't do him in, heart surgery might — any medical expert agreeing he surely wouldn't survive.

If you struck the jackpot, having an exact scenario as I did regarding Mrs. North Shore for your initial haircutting lesson, these are unambiguous and concise directives; follow them rigorously.

We're going to safeguard under lock-and-key her braided semi-spherical mounds, for visiting days at Dr. North Shore's assisted living facility.

✝

BY JEHR SCHIAVO
WRITING AS GERARD SAINT D'ANGELO

✝

ANYBODY CAN DO IT

Gently unwind each cinnamon bun's shape, allowing
these braids to drop from her center parting.

Begin your cutting procedure on dry hair.

Starting from your willing participant's left or right
side, whichever you prefer, this long braid should permit
from the scalp onto braid's inception a minimum of five
to seven inches in unbraided hair.

Carefully raise one braid with the hand not holding
your scissors. You definitely don't under any circumstance
want an accident to happen by slicing into her scalp.

Be so very cautious when you snip the braid off
at its inception; have two elastic ties close by, one for
each, ready to bind — preventing the snipped end from
unbraiding on its own.

If you achieved self-assurance thus far she hasn't any
other choice, she'll have to give up the other braid too,
which you'll remove as well, repeating step/snip one.

There, if you'll be considerate enough, recoil gingerly
each braid back into its tidy braided semi-spherical

mound. Pin, holding its shape securely in place; two separate Ziploc Snack Bags should fit perfectly, traveling wherever she pleases.

You'll be cutting her hair, leaving about the same amount of length required to pin those decorative braids back on when Dr. North Shore's visiting day arrives; by my assessment he won't ever feel or notice any difference.

Mrs. North Shore will use the rear-view and car makeup mirror in her husband's nursing home parking lot — one, two, three, a breeze, attaching both braided semi-spherical mounds, positioned as though they hadn't ever been cut, within those few seconds it took to apply his wife's favorite Chanel lipstick color.

This could be difficult describing what your patron's hair will resemble afterward, but I'll give it a go. After step one, cutting off her braids, you may presume Mrs. North Shore were victim of that brunt insane asylum patient's devious folly when she'd been quite innocently asleep. If your patron pleads and begs, don't show weakness by handing her a mirror; the appearance will look abrupt, as too savage. She'll have heart failure, putting yourself in dire jeopardy when paramedics and police soon arrive to discover incriminating evidence: two Ziploc bags containing Mrs. North Shore's visiting day hairpieces. Your alibi won't make sense to hardened cops; this kitchen which had been yours for cooking and entertaining guests is now their crime scene, cordoned off by yellow tape, a possible homicide. For your own sake reveal her haircut after it's actually been cut properly, not in this garden hedge-trimmer state.

✝

✝

DIRECTOR'S CUT

If I were to select only one haircut so exquisitely practical for every human, females and males covering seven continents, which would seem striking whomever wore it, yet appear a downright different cut on each, I'd pick Jehrcut exhibit A, lesson 1.

It's a classy crowd pleaser, ostensibly having the unique ability to complement any person's consummate bone structure, facial and cranial. Dating back nearly six hundred years in history, our St. Joan of Arc, a perfect representative; calling to mind she allegedly prepared this cut on herself. I should be capable without John Maddenesque scribbling or Keith Haring childish diagrams displaying the theory, while inspiring any valiant soul marching forth to proceed with similar prowess as France's femme fatale.

Twiggy heralded the 1960s fashion eruption; 70s exposed Liza Minnelli; 80s pumped Joan Jett; 90s saw Isabella Rossellini; by this third millennium women's coquette short haircuts have become wildly popular:

Sienna Miller, Emma Watson, and Michelle Williams. Throughout the last fifty years this hairstyle's been transfigured; its characteristics are altered by minor degrees in length, a perimeter's outline consideration.

I wouldn't propose the shortest version; extremely short hair isn't forgiving. Being a precision haircutter will not act as your motive. This immediate goal has more to do with ease reducing vast amounts of length — while sensing what ability feels like, having control, when hairstylists convert another person's image, their patron's out-of-the-ordinary before-and-after difference.

Had your imagination already clicked gears forward, you visualized Mrs. North Shore's upcoming Jehrcut, each and every hair on her head to be approximately four inches in length. At the common rate of growing a half-inch per month, this would've taken any normal person eight months to grow, if it had then been shaved clean, starting out ultramodern. Meaning to say, if you bought any decent electric clipper set, their guards determining exact length all over, your male patron could thankfully sport Sting's crop using a number-eight guard, an equivalent natural growth of two months. Had this happy-go-lucky experiment been shaved clean starting out (seven more weeks worth of growth than Sting), your volunteer replicates Chris Martin's hairstyle; one month longer, *Fight Club* scruffy Brad Pitt.

My creative impression: if the man is balding to such an extent as Jude Law, don't waste time using guard number two, matching Jude's barber; take it right down, premiering your patron's skin — contrast between abundance at his sides and back only accentuates thin sickly hair on top.

The general picture: this classic haircut clipped at those same lengths all over will be tasteful by varying degrees in growth on any given individual, appearing significantly different as well because of distinct textures and specific growth patterns — moreover, our unique faces.

Dame Judi Dench, Sid Vicious, both English, within reason absolutely interchangeable haircuts. Sid's was edgier and longer than Judi's; one combs hers, the other refused to wash his. Each hairstyle iconically their own, prompting clients to download online photographs, bringing a cell phone's saved image into hairstylists worldwide pleading, "Can you make my hair look like this?" Near parallels: Prince Harry's haircut to Halle Berry's archetypal spiky coif. This isn't a revelation, releasing trade secrets; I'm merely giving you encouragement — go ahead, pick up your scissors; we're cutting some hair.

You mustn't try this: we upon occasion see exclusively in cartoons the credulous character's body part, tail usually, getting stuck inside an electrical outlet, every hair stood exaggeratedly on end, directly out from where it grew. When you've finished cutting this is your ultimate objective: you'll need every hair on that head cut the same length from where it grows; finite perimeter details remain discretionary.

Told ya, it's gonna be a cakewalk. Look at your fingers outstretched, you can see they are: pinky, ring finger, middle and index, each about three-quarters of an inch wide, four inches total, not cramming them together, allowing breathing room between each digit — the fleshy guard guiding this haircut's favorable outcome.

Picture nothing else except this: use four fingers to secure not dripping wet but towel-dried hair, keeping pinky, ring and middle digit planted firmly parallel from the scalp, cutting what you'll comb through smoothly, secured by your index finger. Basically what you're doing is creating a three- to four-inch guard around this gutsy person's head; remove any hair protruding past the index finger's guide.

Here's a red blinking STOP sign: pay crucial attention before proceeding, concentrate, remember this cutting implement is extremely sharp; hair won't ever sense anything being cut, fingers do.

Scissors have a straight edge; lines they cut do not coincide with the contour of our skull — heads aren't cubes akin to SpongeBob SquarePants. If you cut across the length of your securing middle and index fingers, you'll discover what stumbling block most stylists ignore, smoothing corners caused by straight lines through conventional cutting — their oversight comparable to well-defined cuts on fabric or paper using scissors.

Your substitution, texturize — it's a term which essentially could be defined by some as deliberate mistakes. Don't cut straight across the inside of your middle and index fingers; rather imagine a serrated edge with its repetitious "v" zigzag formation cutting into hair at forty-

five degree angles. Practice cutting small v's on paper —
your sawtooth line should look as the stegosaurus shape,
tail's tip to puny head, each "v" cut a quarter-inch wide,
connected by diagonals alternating direction.

If there could be a remote opportunity for profuse
hemorrhaging to become reality, why cut anywhere near
your priceless fingers? Keep your scissors' point about
an inch away from those delicate fingers, making then
the final product four inches in length all over, a sexy
moppish pixie — sufficient for Academy Award winner
Anne Hathaway, and Mrs. North Shore.

That wasn't so confusing, was it? Why not take a short
break, let's go off-roading.

✝

✝

GPS

Ikea provides customers with quasi-directions, though
whenever I've been sucked into their vortex, caught up
in the moment, excited about some frivolous product
a Swedish designer keenly believed could sell millions,
I had completely forgotten about past defeated hours
assembling merchandise once at home.

Had you also shopped at Ikea, you've already
found out their diagrams aren't that much assistance
anyway; secondly, no surprise, factories quite often
omit vital parts; third, malfunctioning misaligned
holes, which brought us back frustratedly for exchanges
or returns, locating missing screws, nuts, and bolts,
perhaps all three. Grab a number, can be an hour —
maybe more — waiting. What you'll then discover
without a receipt or not repackaged to their return
clerk's satisfaction: you might be taking whatever
merchandise right back home, though not before
jerry-rigging it on top of your car again — possibly
sticking partially out the hatchback, making this

drive stressful, too, just as that previous trip leaving Ikea's parking lot.

Displayed inside elevators, stairwells, restroom common areas, above automatic shopping cart dispensers, cashiers, or anywhere else this cunning megastore can squeeze available space, you may have noticed the quaint poster of a cute yellow vintage Mini Cooper — maybe it's an Italian 1950s version by Fiat, their Cinquecento — illustrating ease; several Ikea boxes neatly stacked, tied atop, photographed in some Swedish forest, right outside Pippi Longstocking's village.

Drawings and photos will be deceiving; Mr. Haute Coiffure rejects the thought of disappointment. Our haircutting hints in reality necessitate no visual directions whatsoever; there are but two and only these exclusive key paired words composing the science of a haircut: longer or shorter.

Persnickety I'll stay, concerning nearly everything I come in contact with; the energy spent on heads of hair being cut no exception. Telling anyone I'm sickened by bad hair, specifically haircuts, would be way too dramatic. I'll get over someone else's uninspired palate within seconds, contrary to exceptionally gifted Karl Lagerfeld who appears outwardly pompous, cringing in perpetual contempt.

Eminent couture designers — Raf Simons, John Galliano, Hedi Slimane — each bring into being genius masterpieces influenced by why they hired their brilliant design teams — foraging avant-garde oddities within

Moroccan cafés, bars Berlin to Los Angeles, Tokyo subways
and Brooklyn sidewalks; time permitting availability,
most would do it themselves. If it isn't the homeless muse
donning bundled layers of uncoordinated random pants
and overcoats, or an appliquéd motif sweater worn by a
doddering European woman buying provisions at her local
farmer's market — it's those budget-strapped art students,
grabbing whatever's nearest on their floor, then walking
outside, shuffling toward morning coffee.

Inspiration is sporadically met, be it Spanish moss,
rubble during highrise demolition — possibly catastrophic
natural disaster — or most often in my case, haircuts
attempted by that person done themselves — an amateur,
who hadn't the foggiest technical notion what they were
doing. Those cutting their own hair with individuality in
mind should be both applauded and credited.

The pureness of obvious error blended with artistic
intention, for my taste, exceeds any dry bar blowout
on a *Real Housewives* soft-porn-wannabe, role-playing
debauchery weekend in Las Vegas, accompanied by her
dumpy husband. I find no perceptible interest in her,
connecting mental or physical stimulation, mine only pity
stirred on an emotional level. That lifestyle she projects
has an apparent air of shallow meaning; why without
discrepancy she's compelled to portray a sexpot could by
many psychotherapists be considered the larger issue —
averting beauty within.

I for one will much prefer walking the familiar elderly
woman home, at a measure's leisurely pace from our

neighborhood weekly farmer's market; hoping she invites me into her kitchen, savoring yesterday's warmed-up stew, visiting awhile longer, hearing what experiences made this magnificent lady so beautiful.

Spending my days confined inside a typical salon, Tuesday through Saturday, nine each morning until six or seven at night, would have prevented inhaling life — observing people and relationships in their surroundings. Roaming for pleasure through work-related interests allowed absorbing preferences. Swimming across Cala Creta's unspoiled water while catching sight of Lampedusa's jaw-dropping terrain; devouring oysters and mussels, Tomales Bay to Cape Elizabeth; or pulling away from the dock in Lower Manhattan, glancing backward, watching skyscrapers become tiny heading south toward Red Hook; even LA, its human electricity beyond compare.

How many ever pondered another supplemental document, an addendum we would've received along with the birth certificate discharging us from our hospital birthing location, which included beginning-to-end management? Yours for setting away alongside other important papers — birth certificate, social security card, passport, medical documentation, financial records, and insurance policies. Every now and again when feeling slightly helpless, we might casually open our file, locating this nonexistent guide, verifying what year, month, hour or locale we're supposed to be next. Could be useful having those life directional indicators with us, but would stifle me quickly. I don't know about anyone else; for me, there's something straightforward to be said regarding the aspect of authentic, unexpected disclosure.

✝

☩

VS....BS

Sooner or later anyone conscious would've guessed
additional snide comments were overdue — unfairly
some may argue — aimed at the beauty industry's all-
time influential guru — as of 2012 deceased, having lived
twenty-six years longer than me currently. I couldn't
completely let him off the hook, merely attempt to go
easy, avoid beating around bushes, openly nailing matters
how I've perceived them.

    The bricklayer's plans for any foundation's footing
is a critical aspect at construction's start; no brick shall
be askew, lest all others, sideways and above, misalign
increasingly with each row. Architects, engineers, along
with contractors work together, while building inspectors
also complete their jobs every phase of the way —
guaranteeing us a ride without incident pressing 8, 23,
29, or 79 to visit family, friends, doctors, accountants
and lawyers on upper floors. Earthquake, hurricane,
tornado, nor tsunami will topple this structure — broken
windows, flooded lobby and basement perhaps; however,

our architectural marvels, they'll stay put, withstanding the ravages of environmental phenomena.

Small business plans usually don't take several years before operations begin; a concept tickles us mid-February, doors open for many before that calendar year ends. Smarts have a great deal bringing forth success, not to mention serendipity, this plays an important role also.

Way back, in swinging London a go-go, Great Britain burst with art and design; their kooky invasion captured the world's intrigue — Mary Quant, The Who, James Bond, Op Art, and Vidal Sassoon. The moment's appetite ate up Vidal's geometric line — an incipient flimsy business plan came in timely fashion. Lasting a snappy two-decade rule in accomplishment, until Procter & Gamble bought out his name — not for Sassoon's signature look, but another soap brand, more sodium lauryl sulfate, increasing P&G's suds empire.

I wasn't present on Bond Street, London 1963, where and when Vidal chose inscription after cutting his five once-famous fundamental haircuts. His publicist might've better advised Sassoon.

Lazy, quiet September Sunday afternoon, sailing off Martha's Vineyard, your sloop carves that briny Nantucket Sound under glorious puffy cumulus baby blue sky, when the host, an art history professor at RISD, confidently announces, "Peach of a day, wouldn't you agree? *She's* an absolute beaut gliding across these lovely waters."

A redneck hick will have you engaged, standing next

to him with the hood up on his muscle car, gazing into that 426 HEMI engine's hum; he'll lean in, manually tugging its idle three or four revs, then boasting, "Purrs pretty sweet, don't *she?*"

An Atlantic crossing, far up north at a ducky Edinburgh pub, men inside also shout their praise in dense Scottish droll, what that favored putter delivered on St. Andrews' fifteenth hole, "Ah, *she's* the best club I ever held."

Males have such an appreciation of women they'll refer to their prized possessions after them. The art history professor, muscle car aficionado, and Scottish golf pro — each should've been invited as consultants before Vidal sent out his first press release declaring VIP standing, continuing terminology then already fifty years old, today an entire century. Have you ever, in all your born years, heard someone address any female with a fast and true male name? I can't recollect anybody calling Elizabeth, for instance, Mike, Tom, nor Bill. Who of reasonable mind believed using the name Bob, one hundred years ago, alluding to a woman's haircut, certainly didn't consider grammatical function when referring to females; neither did Sassoon, staking historic proclamation. Whoever she was, even in Vidal's peaking hour, must've hesitated before asking her stylist for a "bob," not to mention nowadays.

Those three non-hairstylists extolling the inherent merit of women come across as gentlemanly in comparison to that cockney crew, handpicked by unformed Sassoon; he and his "roit bench e 'ooligans" simply cleaned up, dressed wearing skinny three-piece shark skin suits. You can hoist any boy from London's East End, he'll though forever be street savvy; I dodged Ozone Park fifty years ago — same difference, still exerting an upfront New York attitude, odds are, always will.

Christening his extensively-known woman's haircut with a masculine name is inconsequential. I will from first-hand experience, while under Vidal's original founding minion, convey what in fact were everyday common occurrences before Sassoon found himself stripped of all his salons, sold cheap to the Regis Corporation, catering business toward downmarket shopping malls.

When a Vidal Sassoon client periodically displayed timid character upon being made aware copious amounts of her hair would soon be removed, she — fleetingly felt apprehensive, generally uneasy — at times started tearing; the styling chair then instantly turned away from that stylist's mirrored station, dismissing this appointment — "go on ahead, get yourself changed, thank you very much" — an impatient stylist walked briskly toward reception, lastly, voided out their patron's pink receipt. Those were the sensitive stylists on a kind day informing their anxious unchartered Vidal Sassoon clients of plans to reduce substantial length. Another Sassoon droid's client, once shampooed, conditioned and reseated for her cut, by different chairside manner, without forewarning during consultation, went straight into emotional shock she did, feeling shears produce a line of arrant severity across the nape's skin; bob, step one, "head down" — other than that she'd been told little else.

The best haircut technicians I've ever observed were those directly imported from Sassoon's inaugural London salons — flawless and robotic, human cutting machines, precision unsurpassed, to a thirty-second of an inch. Training there on Grant Avenue in San Francisco for me during that period was the end of an era — Vidal's army hadn't yet split up; his soldiers were still positioned.

Any patron allowing herself to break down crying before several surrounding clients and their stylists throughout the cutting room's reflective mirrors — an infrequent situation, gawking upon which was not above anyone's gravitas. The Vidal Sassoon clientele we served wasn't regarded as much more than a number, an extension of our pink receipt listing services and products with corresponding boxes to check off. Without her, who would carry it from reception after donning a mocha cotton smock? Forty-five minutes later, perhaps three hours depending on services rendered, powdered any stray hairs before changing as revenue was then due.

Geometrics, wow man, groovy. When Vidal, in his salad days, laid business brick and mortar, everything mod moved him — unfortunately this was narrow-minded; a subtle effect hadn't its place accessorizing fashion of the early 1960s. Graduated bob, box bob, A-line bob, layered bob — a bob's a bob. Very difficult, nearly impossible, to achieve proper cutting's greatness utilizing Sassoon's hard line pressed against a woman's graceful neck. Any bob creates bluntness upon a woman's soft curvaceous skin, harshly framing milky smooth facial features, evoking an object pasted on — hers, another Vidal Sassoon haircut, his wiggish hat.

Zero blending, hair upon skin — none whatsoever, differentiation between both explicitly black-and-white; ultra-happening wearing luscious false eyelashes, Nancy Sinatra white boots, hot pink patent leather mini skirt, only to fade away years before Jagger and Richards' masterful *Let it Bleed*, challenged thereafter by the Beatles' sappy farewell ditty, *Let it Be*.

Vidal's chain housing automaton cutters spread out dotting continents, while clients eventually became accustomed, quoting many here, to their "lesbian haircuts," including the Duke of Bedford's reference toward his wife's Sassoon cut. Vidal's insistence: he, liberating women, permitted their continuance living — less wave lotion, rollers, hood dryer, backcombing, hairspray, and/or lacquer prior to his arrival. Mr. Haute Coiffure and I both stand solidly convicted women stay to this day enslaved by the renamed trappings Sassoon formally introduced over six decades ago: mousse, gel, protector spray, blow dryer, electric hot iron, brush for intense heat, completing his look with finishing spray, a mild lacquer. Come on, honestly, Vidal didn't offer that much progress, did he?

About Sassoon's so-called modifications: I've wondered if patronizing Antoine of Paris, star previous to Vidal, might've been a more fulfilling two hours for clientele, pampered in the mode women should be, opposing Vidal's half-century and counting residual theory — daily barbaric wrestling matches, tugging hair into every which direction, diminishing its elasticity, burning, using direct heat, continued repudiating with great effort, her morning submission ritual complete. Does a woman desire to be told what she must do? An imbecile who'd woken from the Dark Ages can inform anybody that correct answer; why then would she treat her hair by such cruel methods each day, as senseless thugs bashing one another for no apparent reason?

✝

SWINE

Those professionals still breathing within the beauty
industry who've rested their careers on Sassoon's grossly
inflated general estimation: show yourself, step right up
if you will, whether at all possible to take time off, away
from your salon hawking every destructive service between
Brazilian blowout and Japanese digital perm, shrieking in
Vidal's defense, "but he did, I insist — Vidal Sassoon freed
women, no longer subjugated under beauty's yoke."

Speak to us, oh tenured company stylist, director,
artistic director, senior artistic director, international
artistic director — whichever elaborate job description was
yours — about when you were summoned without pay to
Vidal's hotel suite — in town for his annual staff meeting,
there blow drying ex-wife Beverly before their evening
out, she herself too work-shy or incapable, possibly
both, evidently beneath her husband; besides he'd been
tremendously overwhelmed, handling personally those
affairs at your once-beloved salon, dedicating a whole
fifty-five minutes per year. Were you also in attendance

soon thereafter, during those annual meetings when Sassoon stalked through that salon beforehand, scarcely acknowledging anyone, passing gesture to loyal emigrant employees; striding without interruption, as stunned clientele who hadn't blinked observed Vidal whisked toward your former manager's office?

During my closing teenage year I witnessed this very key night's events unfolding, standing at strict attention among others who believed probable another paycheck beyond Vidal's visit. A white glove week it was prior to our monarch's entrance — scrubbed and polished an entire salon's surface, receiving then its mephitic layer of paint. Staff were prepped accordingly; receptionists, I'm positive, not actually instructed how they should genuflect — somehow, though, given clear orders what his eminence closely expected, their bowing curtsey.

His timing, impeccable, arriving approximately thirty minutes after all five o'clock appointments arrived, our last for that day seated, well underway receiving their haircuts, having already been shampooed. Cold fear penetrated pretty much every staff member — maids, receptionists, assistants, stylists, and management, to such an extent in density only a chainsaw might've found resolution; heaven forbid I extend my hand, "Hello, Sir, it's an honor."

Difficult twenty minutes to deal with — receptionists finalizing that day's receipts, speedier stylists packing equipment, others frantic, desperately getting clients done before the clock struck 6:15 p.m., promptly adjourning toward our gallows. Innocent and

mischievous, couldn't to save my life piece together why
everyone was behaving so uncharacteristically; not one
stylist discussed drinks at the Iron Horse on Maiden
Lane following our staff meeting, or much else. I was
baffled, why such a solemn affair?

Through the intercom meant to announce client
arrivals came a different serious tone above our heads —
hearing then management order all upper staff members
downstairs immediately. Single file, none excitedly
shoving; those previously exposed to Vidal hushed
comments distasteful in sentiment, hoping he would be
quick. Not me — first encounter with history; I went
forward, jockeying a choice seat, while veteran stylists
glued themselves to the back wall; slowly more began
appearing, dragging resistant footsteps.

Front row, far right side, aisle seat, Vidal's immediate
left — the only feasible way his royal highness could've
missed my glowing smile's eager intent was if he were
Ray Charles. Not yet fully formed Mr. Haute Coiffure,
a sole staff member in Sassoon's presence imbuing
star-struck idolized euphoria, he then occupying the
haircutting wizard's throne feet away, this protégé
was awestruck, perceptible delight written all over my
face. When the last available folding chair had been
taken, every movement ceased, accompanied by pin
dropping silence. Sassoon commenced pace inches
before me, halting momentarily; we stared into each
other, Vidal then landed a stinging palm across my
cheek, inquiring aloud, "and what exactly do you find so

amusing, Son?" A strange tingling sensation instantly ran up my temperature, rising cauldron bubbly hot, while simultaneously freezing like glacier ice, altering exhilaration into utter embarrassment.

Sassoon's lecture hadn't any finesse, nothing of pleasantries; beyond Vidal's strike, I heard his sharpness within seconds — informing us he preferred not to delay guests elsewhere, our meeting would be brief. Using both hands with the same force as his projected voice, he barked our salon services brought in the worst numbers out of all his salons, having declined terribly, more so than that previous year. Concluded, if figures didn't increase by our building a stronger client base we'd be rapidly seeking new employment. Vidal clearly lost his forbearance — if anybody should bold-face lie, expressing he ever had control in disposition to begin with. He finished talking down at us in under fifteen minutes; however, not without lastly including, "My products are holding this salon up, I don't need you."

Writing by first-hand knowledge concerning issues specifically within the beauty industry is my intention. Dealings of Sassoon's hapless personal life — decisions other than salons or products — are well-recognized for those curious; suffice saying neither emotional comfort nor satisfaction seemingly reached Vidal into his cushy retirement.

At day's close I don't deny Sassoon, alongside artistic underlings, cut precise lines; categorically he and team should be credited. Fraudulent could be too

disagreeable a word, but I'm stumped replacing such
with an appropriate term defining Vidal's purported
revolutionizing the beauty industry, liberating women.
Part and parcel, two principal arguments I submit Vidal
was artful at deception: firstly, every classic Sassoon
haircut required chemically-based styling products, blow
dryer, along with irons — virtual perfection appropriate
for archival photographic purposes, however, absolutely
impossible for her home replication. Secondly, Vidal's
kingdom of clients' hair was not remotely healthy as
he faithfully professed. A finished Sassoon haircut
necessitates sectioning hair into four parts: quarter-
to half-inch methodical sections, ingrained as basic
practice — blow drying can take trained assistants twenty
minutes, their assigned proficient stylist ten, clients at
home thirty, others an hour, perhaps more.

Any professional blow dryer's heat set at high, which
is imperative achieving what Sassoonites clarify by
instruction as "a finished look," should cause anybody
to blurt out one of two four-letter words, often both,
when inevitably skin contact accidents occur — three-
hundred-and-ninety-five-plus degrees, scalding air,
burning flesh. I wouldn't ask just anyone to experiment
with their own skin patch test. Between wrist and elbow,
top of our masochist's forearm, they shall for funsies
turn on this egregious blow dryer, blasting steady heat
exactly the distance used to dry hair, a few inches away,
twenty minutes every day, directly onto their arm's bare
skin. An approximate interval from one haircut until its

next should be about two months; that's the period of weeks we'll permit this masochist their enjoyment. Any takers — would anyone supervise examination of the dermatological injury inflicted by stupidity, decided eight weeks earlier?

When damaged, wet hair is completely misleading, having the appearance of healthy tresses. Blown out and/or ironed, burning shut, seals the hair's outside cuticle layer, producing by all means "a finished look" — however, having brief glassy results.

In fact-checking certain dates, my absolute earthly everything Jeanette relayed diverse quotes, which Vidal either came up with by himself or responded to questioning through interviews. Not a person who's ever heard the name Sassoon can deny notoriety; his, eternally synonymous with hair, he gained obvious triumph, perceived as an adored expert. There is one particular laughable phrase of Sassoon quotations that interested me. I can hear Vidal in his dreamy, supremely marketable British accent, touting a wicked quote so conclusively false; Jeanette determined this selection from various pages exposing other fibs. Vidal Sassoon sold premeditated trickery, stating, "Hair must be in tip-top shape"; a precision haircut would leave it "looking marvelous, having bounce by just one flick of the comb."

For the record, Sassoon was in no way, shape, or form responsible for Mia Farrow's haircut before shooting *Rosemary's Baby*; she did it herself using fingernail scissors before one of Vidal's lackeys attempted to fine-tune what had already been her personal handiwork's *pièce de résistance*. Farrow later revealed Vidal had nothing to do with her pixie style, further saying Roman Polanski brokered a deal, paying Sassoon for this prized charlatan haircutting publicity stunt.

It is true no hairstylist alive wasn't directly influenced by Sassoon; neither were any clients we've rendered haircuts for. Since I've presented the case that his alleged honorable name, bearing wash and wear thinking, be challenged, there was no alternate way around it. With indubitable respect to precision haircutting's innovator, he'd but gone only a portion of the distance.

✟

✝

CORNER OF FACT AND FICTION

Even though I could barely decipher legibility by any physician, at the end of routine check-ups — maybe I'd suddenly experienced flu ailments or persistent pain — doctors inevitably hand over their higgledy-piggledy handwritten prescription. I listened attentively hearing directions to take whatever this was however many times daily, before or after meals, for whichever amount of days they instructed me. Almost felt healed being handed the five-inch white paper square imparting a printing press' intelligible generic font, this doctor's name, accredited degree, address and telephone number.

Somehow our pharmacist must've also been educated in the expertise of reading most every physician's sloppy handwriting. Didn't much matter to me, the way I viewed my situation — A) seriously needed this medication; B) implicitly trusted both, doctor and druggist, their professional peak standard normally of utmost combined ranking. This relationship, physician to pharmacist, is tight as any separate entities can possibly

be; legally, they function together seamlessly. On occasion
the druggist made a few inquiries before issuing powerful
narcotics, when we'd then likely overhear verification
by this pharmacy phoning our doctor's office. Prior
to paying this stern pharmacist, they'd reiterate how
much and when, echoing what the doctor had told us,
regarding administration of our medication, seeing those
instructions clearly now typed out on that plastic amber
bottle's directions.

The Food and Drug Administration mandates each
and every ingredient contained in all retail bottles
(beauty products included) be plainly itemized.
Unless we ourselves are scholared chemists, the most
understandable ingredient is water, followed by
several unpronounceable names, which also appear on
many other product labels. FDA law requires listing a
manufacturer's ingredients not alphabetically, but by
order of largest quantity per unit.

Markup on a bottle of shampoo or conditioner can
be astronomical. The FDA doesn't control pricing —
captains of industry do; some consumers are willing
to pay $150 each for ritzy eight-ounce shampoo and
conditioner bottles. Unless a prescription for an
iniquitous $300 shampoo and conditioner combo comes
from your physician to be filled at the neighborhood
pharmacy, you've been conned by some naughty
hairstylist, this money better spent elsewhere.

Many health nuts don't mind shelling out $10 or more
for a lousy liter of mineral water; they'll stay hydrated

before arriving at their fitness center ready to collect two warm, fluffy towels. I'd lay even money they carry inside their sports bag at least two eight-ounce beauty product bottles, packaging worth nickels each, together filled with $50 of retail liquid, containing mostly water — although probably not from the Swiss Alps. Why should Switzerland bother messing about bottling hair detergent along with cream rinse, given their already superior operation — bottles mere pennies, water practically nothing, nominal cost for shipping and handling; they still make out like bandits.

Once and far ago in a sincere hamlet, shoppers would walk into the local apothecary's domain. Honorable retailers in storyville's earlier times were those where buyers should shop these days, knowing within reason they're purchasing excellent-grade merchandise at fair economical pricing.

Why Mr. Haute Coiffure, have you formed additional opinionated inferences again?

"Good day, might I be of any assistance? Yes, 'tis truly delightful this spring. My Missus told me you're taking summer holiday on Corsica; do dress snug for that ship's voyage, evenings especially can remain somewhat nippy you know, ah such a marvelous journey the whole family will forever look back holding dear."

Lazy pace, won't you, inside an honest apothecary, betwixt their frequently experienced dangling brass bell at the proprietor's front door announcing visitor's entry, to that homey rhythm made as your leather boots

meander across waxed oak flooring; a hickory ladder
on rolling track, aid for lofty cabinetry, surrounded by
ebony wainscot paneled walls, yet each and every item
well-lit behind pristine curved display cases, having glass-
beveled-prism edges; once inside throughout its entirety,
we could not be served anywhere from more competent
hands this very day.

Depending how many centuries we'd travel back
encircling the Mediterranean Sea, all things into
consideration, Mr. Haute Coiffure wouldn't alter much
among those old-world products available through each
region's apothecarist. Had those goods been sold today,
luxury retailers undoubtedly couldn't wait, clamoring for
exclusive rights; the novelty of packaging sans complexities
would spark Fifth Avenue's feeding frenzy. A definite
fad following this millennium's beginning, easily spotted
inside trendy Williamsburg or Venice Beach stores,
purveyors selling boutiquesque beauty products. An
interior designer's aesthetics also thoroughly intoxicated
by this era, installing timeless small white octagon tiles
throughout each chain store's scheduled roll-out, before
you know it covering the earth's ends.

What corporate faux heirloom boutiques miss
are two important elements: natural aging through
hundreds of years, and the more significant point:
that well-thought-out guidance given behind curved
glass counters attending our ancestry from current
generation to their children's children. What you
then provided for your dedicated customers brought

about different meaning; this was the apothecarist family's future reputation, either in jeopardy offering inferior merchandise or remaining resolute, poised by great-grandfather and wife's tested knowledge from previous generations. Rest assured, inside this nostalgic apothecary in the South of France or any moderately populated Greek island, we'd not today see such pared down shampoo and conditioner selections; dissimilar to these days, seeing stockpiles developed from sought-after brands.

Entire aisles — both sides — at supermarket, chain drugstore, mega-mart, or beauty supply, offering every shampoo-conditioner combo known and then some, containing enough chemicals, the back identifying ingredient enumeration requiring a sizeable bit, informing what few of us comprehend. Should a present-day customer be confused, they'll ask an employee, typically uninformed, earning minimum-wage salary, biding the hours away, hopefully returning home before their children's bedtime (if they have kids).

Perhaps another consumer gathered information from an ad on television, other instances flipping through magazines, could've been celebrity endorsements, maybe not; was that authentic gorgeous hair we'd seen, or computer-generated special effects? Duped exactly as publicly traded companies aim, justifying hundreds of billions spent nationally and globally, hoaxing Silly Jilly alongside Willy during quarterly print in conjunction with TV ad campaigns.

Within that vignette's yesteryear flash, shopkeeper knew what order customers desired before walking in. They had sold to your family a double-fist block of pure olive oil soap every third week the past sixteen years. You used it, so did your spouse, including two daughters, eight, another twelve, three sons, six, ten, and fourteen. Store-wrapped, by paper made from wood pulp and ordinary twine; the olive oil block itself wasn't at all ornate. For a while an etched emblem of two branch sprigs and attached olives presented themselves — solid soap such as that, a dozen uses only begins to dissolve its logo's past embossed imagery. Seven family members living inside that household: father, slightly dark complexion, having thick salt-and-pepper curls; mother, fair skin, straight sandy-blonde hair; their kids, each partially sharing both parents' distinguished features. On that same visit picking up the block of olive oil soap, someone, usually Mother, also purchased a corked, sturdy glass half-pint bottle, containing pure plant-derived oil.

Seems the whole village also has a natural beauty about them; their hair and skin have an unexpected glistening excellence. If you asked anyone what they cleansed and moisturized their skin with they'd tell us that tantamount answer — inquiring, how did everybody there get so blessed having such beautiful hair?

✝

✝

Shampoo-Poo

Mr. Haute Coiffure isn't equipped to go up against Estée Lauder, Revlon, nor Unilever — would've included L'Oréal and Procter & Gamble as examples, but they've already received more acknowledgment than they deserve throughout earlier pages. Under these monolithic umbrellas, such companies purchase famous names, building their brand yet bigger, commanding unstoppable compounded fiscal cash flow; they're not going anywhere. Same with GM or Toyota, doesn't appear to make any difference whatsoever how many recalls consumers receive. Cars are necessary; unfortunately, buyers place confidence in nefarious auto manufacturers who've proven time and again otherwise. Most consider Toyota the industry leader of fuel-efficient automobiles; we have also come to understand drivers will continue purchasing those cars at top dollar, despite additional precious cost, risking their lives alongside passengers' personal safety and, God forbid, mortality.

Shampoos and conditioners in our civilized society are well-appreciated; although recognized popular products, following that company's explicit directions to a T, completely damage hair, while leaving offensive fragrances long after thorough rinsing — Aveda being only one example, heisting absurd amounts at the retail counter.

From professional and personal experience within my industry, this beautifier obtained practical knowledge, however, scientific engineering through corporate funding has obliterated centuries of hair and skin purity. Selfish desires — random acquisitions have reached unfair business practice status by every sense of the expression — case in point, Roxanne Quimby and Clorox swindling Burt's Bees from Burt Shavitz. Promoting evolution of inner beauty became similar to climbing up the downward escalator, buyers going nowhere fast.

In the proximity of listed ingredients, above or below, to either side, on every shampoo bottle are those company's specific directions. If I were über gung-ho, perhaps I'd research that shrewd person who first devised labeling directions; what words we read isn't anything of the sort.

How to shampoo hair has thus far been clearly noted on any bottle I've seen. Frankly, every shampoo bottle's directions I've ever examined has more emphasis on how frequent shampooing must occur than proper shampooing itself.

Other than Mr. Haute Coiffure, somebody else must have at least once said to themselves, "I don't need a shampoo every day; why are they force-feeding me this stuff?"

"What do those people mean, 'repeat if necessary'; should that additional application be repeated for any apparent reason I'm not grasping?"

Who doesn't occasionally have condescending flavor? I will mind my Ps and Qs until that certain nanosecond when all damnation breaks loose, refusing no longer, holding back an acute tongue. Are not gouging excessively high profits per unit sufficient? Hadn't some abashed beauty CEO at any instant halted, born having conscience, been pinched by their own compunction concerning ethics? Why insult the consumer's intelligence another moment more? Beauty companies are not actually instructing users with mere directions; they also provide a subliminal tactic, having customers quickly use unnecessary additional product so they'll buy more bottles quicker. Don't bet the farm on it; no turn of events soon will you see any product company changing their shampoo bottle's directions.

A man wielding some noisy jackhammer resurfacing our roadways needs that grubby hair shampooed each night following backbreaking hours; his roofer pal would benefit from doing the same. My women patrons often object, "But Jehr, I'm working out at the gym on a daily basis." Nope, I disagree, not even close to being true, this is perspiration, not dirt; she — and men for that matter — remembers what she'd seen printed on the back of misleading shampoo bottles.

Jacqueline Kennedy Onassis — America lauded
her, a class above as could possibly be. She, without
doubt cancelled out being waited on hand and foot at
every instant by her utter poise — elegance, such grace
exemplified, especially defined under extraordinary severe
circumstance as any one person should not ever witness.
Wherever Jackie was, her peculiar fetish followed; for
what she endured, I believe such pampering really an
honor on behalf of each chambermaid, who served this
once-in-a-lifetime stars and stripes royal. Before an
evening's sleep or her fifty-minute mid-afternoon beauty
nap, Jackie expected a complete, newly washed and lightly
ironed set of D. Porthault linens on this bed upon which
she was about to recline. Although there couldn't be any
better method for every square inch of my body realizing
sweet dreams would suddenly arrive, common sense
should also inform me that somebody's buying way too
many expensive sheets around this penthouse. If Jackie
had only one set of sheets, those were potentially washed
seven hundred thirty times annually, not hardly. She
undoubtedly had a slew of sets, consuming some fortunate
staff member's hours, constantly ordering brand spanking
new ones — Egyptian, Martian from Mars, whatever type,
in the highest thread-count available; still couldn't handle
that much abuse, fabric softener can do so much.

I'll challenge anyone alive to come straight out telling
a big fat lie, "I have an extra head of hair; I've plenty
more stored, piled inside my attic, basement and garage,
leave me alone, I'd shampoo twice daily just like Jackie

O washed her sheets if I'm in the mood." Certainly, do whatever floats your boat; but remember perspiration by overheating is simply water — how much industrial fallout could one head of hair attract on a given day? Probably less dust than Jackie's sheets collected while catching her midday cat-nap.

After performing my craft enough years I noticed a common trait among clientele commissioning me. Usually, prior to my arrival at their place, if that were the situation, they would have recently shampooed. Should my pop-up space be an option for this willing subject, they'll make the trip to me, typically understanding a shampoo basin isn't available, having already shampooed their hair earlier at home. Much the same as how most excessively brush, being extra careful prior to dental appointments; out of courtesy for our dentist and their hygienist, we're conscious about bringing leftover breakfast or lunch between teeth.

Won't ever cease to amaze me, an explanation seems almost always necessary describing what clients have done incorrectly — washed hair during a shampoo, rather than properly cleansing the sebaceous oil at their scalp. An expression I'll inevitably discover on their face is no different from my own the first time I'd ever heard a dentist instruct I should brush in circular rotating movements, instead of brushing up and down. Plaque built by improper brushing vanished during that dental exam, as did whatever morsels missed from vigorous, wrongful vertical motion.

Not knowing within absolute certainty — traveling to them, or alternatively frequenting my unsalon — because their hair had by then already dried, I would often gently inquire, "When did you shampoo last?" Without fail patrons respond, "Just before you got here," or they coming to me, "This morning when I took a shower." Many clients I hadn't seen before didn't remove their scalp's sebaceous oil; the hair itself was clean, but, from shampooing by ineffective habitual manner, theirs became dull and fuzzy. Our hair's texture is sensitive as silk, not car tires requiring an occasional scrub. These, by the way, were those clients complaining their hair gets oily overnight — "Come morning I'll have to shampoo; I'm not leaving my house if I don't."

Splendid, an honest-to-goodness piece of advice from Mr. Haute Coiffure: don't during any shampoo ever actually wash your hair. Use instead the fingers' padded tips, ten little Indians forming a sebaceous oil dance over and around your scalp. If you're from that squeak test school, check your root area, not the hair's shaft. Hair itself will be cleansed sufficiently through appropriate rinsing, removing any micro particles and pollution. After granting water its full rinsing potential your head will become clean as a whistle.

✝

✝

CRÈME DE LA CRÈME

Think about prematurely throwing a batch of laundry into your dryer before the washer's rinse cycle had been finished. Residual detergent on that load would then come out thirty tumble-dried minutes later crunchy, coarse, and drab, similar to hair having been conditioned with shampoo traces remaining. Every washer has its final cycle; too often I'm impatient, hurried, opening while on spin, tossing everything into my dryer — no actual physical harm there, but yes, disadvantageous conditioning hair before the shampoo process is complete.

There is a laundry comparison. Before applying conditioner, for satisfactory results, excess water needs to be thoroughly squeezed out after rinsing; that's your pre-conditioning spin cycle.

The sopping wet sponge cannot absorb more moisture; neither will hair thirsty for its daily conditioning dose still full of water.

A correct conditioning application is opposite of shampooing. Focus your conditioning attention on nourishing that hair's shaft, massaging single-downward movements onto hair, avoiding the scalp; accompanied by a wide-tooth comb furthering assistance, distributing conditioner evenly, fastening longer hair upward if necessary prior to rinsing.

Those very last minutes showering, after conditioner absorbs into your hair for a while — you'd been soaping up, perhaps shaving — this is then the proper time to rinse, not seconds following application.

Lean your head back, permitting the shower pressure to rinse until water runs and feels clear. Don't allow any conditioner to remain. You'll know when it's thoroughly removed; if not, hair appears to require another shampoo, defeating your daily routine's purpose.

Fortunately, there is no such thing as the hair police. Breaking rules can be somewhat exciting, most everyone does it — seeing how much we might get away with without getting caught. I used to cheat eating pizza, pasta, dense crusty bread with butter, pastries, ice cream even doughnuts — they were enjoyable too — maple bars or crumb cake particularly, although none agreed with my waistline, nor cancer catching me in the form of a melanoma tumor. All these alongside other highly processed foods contain scarce or no nutritional value, empty calories metabolising into sugar once inside our body, enriching cancer's growth. Hair is one of those fallen-to-the-wayside aspects in our lives, different than, say, putting on an unwanted thirty pounds, which could with due diligence shed; thinning hair hardly ever reverts direction to its previous density.

It isn't imperative to make appointments at the beauty salon for those periodic chemical services; prolonged meetings there damaging hair promote alopecia, where previously boasting substantially more, thinning can also easily happen through poor homecare. Over-shampooing, meaning every day, sometimes twice, rubbing hair on top of the head in a wad with both palms, incomplete rinsing, not squeezing excess water out before conditioning, perhaps none at all, maybe half-hearted attempts — one unkind day abnormal hair loss will indeed present itself. We don't really need a stylist ruining hair; clients wreak havoc on it themselves, unfortunately, even those uncooperative subsequent to informing them.

Here's an excuse why busy people trying to schedule overcrowded lives, despite being advised, dismiss allocating enough minutes in a day for themselves, those who barely make it into their morning shower. A spouse on their way outdoors, another somewhere inside yelling, "Gotta go honey, call you when I get to work — darn it, better hop in the shower, I'm already twenty minutes late." What would have been a pleasant morning ceremony seldom will be, which, remaining plausibly accurate, is why some exploitative beauty industry Einstein contrived shampoo and conditioner within one asinine bottle.

Any normal person can verify there aren't enough hours in a given day to accomplish everything that those center their attention on. Is anyone other than myself willing under oath to make this statement? "Bottles of 2-in-1 shampoo/conditioner won't save much time, nor is the best solution for consistent healthy hair." At this very moment, an average American woman has about three brands of shampoo and conditioner in her shower — she's flummoxed, with every reason to be; the marketplace is downright oversaturated. I'm comfortable endorsing a brush that works effectively toward its goal for every hair type; on the other hand, shampoos along with conditioners to date morphed into some chaotic hodgepodge of scented Tweedledee and Tweedledum products.

A question many might ask themselves sixteen years into this third millennium: "Now that I'm out of my shower with clean, conditioned hair, how can I actually save time?" Life was already crammed with abundant bogus mid-twentieth-century ideas devised by the beauty industry; not only are there more deleterious services offered these days, but prices receiving most any of them and accompanying products soar every year as well.

✝

☩

HOMOGENY

Some time ago I watched a woman walking, late thirties probably, bottle number xyz blonde hair, cut bluntly to the middle of her back, blown dry stick-straight. She appeared superficial and behind the curve, so much I didn't actually see her; this woman's head seemed as though it floated down Third Street, suspended in a time warp, right outside San Francisco's Museum of Modern Art. It, rather her head of hair, could've been on exhibition inside MOMA near Michael Jackson and Bubbles — hers is a concept Jeff Koons ought to earnestly ponder.

The bad-news crier isn't often a welcome party guest; however, truth be told, bottle number xyz blonde hair, cut bluntly to the middle of any woman's back, blown dry stick-straight, won't make her imperfect life any more exemplary, striving for external beauty as she does. I realized long ago offering hairstyles which gave clients pause, having to obsess about their hair was a waste of time, theirs and mine. Behind your knees, at the back of each leg, are their respective bending creases; I elected that area on our body as a barometer. When was your last concern you had about this specific portion — likely, not recently. That was the gold standard Mr. Haute Coiffure set for a patron's hairstyle; if they had to evaluate their hair once between Jehrcuts, I'd not in my perception been effective delivering chic, effortless, healthy, sustainable twenty-first-century hair. When a client has to think about their hair much more than that crease at the back of either leg, something, I believe, must be wrong.

Why would anyone want to worry about it — including me, if I had hair of my own? Whoever has an extra thirty minutes hanging around each morning fussing over hair after showering becomes accustomed to squandering valuable minutes. One hundred eighty-two hours each year, an inordinate measure spent styling one's hair — pardon my harsh criticism, but in all sincerity, get a life. Four considerations: either this person can't quite wrap their mind around how they appear without fantasy; maybe life became a bore, having nothing pressing going on; perhaps desiring another diversion to shirk meaningful obligations; or lastly, didn't have any better alternatives.

When the chips got stacked higher post-Y2K, people essentially went berserk, while all along many were mistakenly under a common assumption this was technology predicted to go thoroughly haywire, our grid allegedly gone squiffy. I was then, and continue to exist, a believer having faith; positive energy will prevail from any deplorable slump. Eventually healthcare and education among other neglected domestic infrastructure will soon be returning in vogue. America's current tendency handling affairs, slighting taxpayers, should also grow tiring — storing Congress, alongside their snail-crawl lawmaking ability, somewhere inside the Smithsonian — another museum, a different antiquated notion as that blown-out xyz blonde on Third Street.

Not all embrace change so very easily; we familiarize ourselves with particular habits, no matter how time-consuming or financially unsound. For an individual exhausting thirty minutes a day, married to that passé, half-century-old Vidal Sassoon concept of slaving over hair, can't fathom towel blotting after showering; bingo, badda bing, badda boom, that's it — reasoning: the haircut enabling her doing so wasn't present.

✝

BY JEHR SCHIAVO
WRITING AS GERARD SAINT D'ANGELO

✝

IT'S THE LIFE

Forgot to mention I was with Jeanette and LouLou
recently in front of SFMOMA, before visiting Roberta,
LouLou's surrogate nonna, hers the same age my mother
would've been if she were alive; Jean's spirit drifted
into heaven twelve years ago at seventy-nine. I'd known
Roberta on-and-off throughout my years living in San
Francisco; I wasn't aware she'd become substitute family
those thirty years earlier while making alterations for my
clothing, though she did, especially after meeting Jeanette
and LouLou. Roberta immigrated to San Francisco from
Lucca, Italy in 1964; I have no delusions she was mod
nor hip back then.

During our last visit Roberta quivered, seeming
exceptionally pale, however, opened an envelope her
fifty-nine year old nephew from Lucca sent containing
a photograph he had enlarged for his aunt to keep.
Roberta's weakened vision had since prevented any
further sewing of alterations, mine or customers',
although she managed to bake the tastiest almond biscotti

we've ever tried. Roberta didn't survive long enough
for our next bi-monthly visit to her flat. The photo was
snapped on vacation in 1984 outside her sister's country
home near Lucca. Several family members were pictured,
including Roberta, eating and drinking lunch al fresco —
the only relative still living, her nephew.

We got along easily because the four of us tended
to agree. She held the enlargement, handed it first to
me, then Jeanette and LouLou — didn't herself let go
after showing us, kept staring at loss, loving voices gone,
welling over Roberta wept, shaking her head. By such
few words of proper English she'd spoken, Roberta was
stunned, communicating how swiftly a life hers had
vanished. I distracted Roberta from her inattentiveness,
painfully missing those deceased, sidetracked our tense
silence by commenting, "There's no better means of
relishing life than being with those we care about, sharing
a meal outside in the fresh air."

Roberta's soul, hers, pure unsullied beauty; she wanted
to feed us with nothing in return, other than our brief
visits. Jeanette didn't email her; Roberta hadn't owned
a computer, though she did have an ordinary landline
telephone — they spoke regularly. She wrote out greeting
cards exactly the way she'd sound those words when
speaking; her blurred sight skipped letters, while every
line had a gradual degree increase in slanted slope.

Discovered something else that afternoon beyond her
'84 trip to Lucca and the grief she expertly hid inside. I
hadn't once over the course of thirty years inquired nor

thought about who cut Roberta's hair. She lived in the
remnants of what was North Beach's formerly thriving
Italian neighborhood. I took for granted that she'd
probably seen the same hairdresser in a discreet, old-
school holdout beauty parlor. Before leaving Roberta
told us she hadn't been to a professional hairstylist since
she left Italy forty-six years ago; by then in Roberta's
final years nearly blind, this captivating woman had been
cutting her own hair.

✟

Gladiator Alley

Rome made a tremendous impact on me, one city in which, I quickly figured, if getting acquainted with at any great length was an issue, I'd need to seek seasonal employment; having not been within the same confines of another's salon in over twenty years didn't matter.

My Near Eastern-born hostess who established herself in Rome hadn't ever touched one client other than a pair of air kisses at each cheek for those clientele who'd come to see her more able staff. She honed her social skills owning the salon, by then forty years; Lisette knew what made people tick, both clients and hairstylists.

Ours was a doomed professional relationship, starting with special preparation prior to my engagement — brought into being entirely on Lisette's part, without question rubbing her stylists the wrong way. They'd been working for Lisette decades themselves; none appreciated so immensely as I had this preferential treatment.

An interior spiral stairway led clients to the beauty salon below her Via Sistina ground-level boutique,

directly across from Valentino's couture palazzo.
Breathtaking views just outside atop the Spanish Steps
and Hassler Villa Medici Hotel, a haven for wealth's
fabulous filthy rich alongside sprinkled aristocracy,
Lisette's next door neighbors.

Many Romans seem rationalized with categorical
determination to emanate superiority — an attitude
understandable for some commoners: plainly, hire a
tourist minivan, ride soaking up Rome, see the Eternal
City yourself, better yet walk. Nothing different if it
were me sent out before dinner at seven years old to
buy handmade ravioli and Pecorino Romano for grating
upon Jean's request. I watched as kids dashed down
narrow cobblestone sidewalks adjacent to Fontana
di Trevi, hearing other young children holler, playing
outside their antecedent's neo-Classical apartment
buildings on Piazza del Pantheon. Teenage students
before or after school, maybe on recess, crowding cafes,
alimentaris and gelaterias nearby. Antica Roma, Basilica
di San Pietro in Vaticano, Roma's Colosseo — let's
face it, these adults who grew from diapers surrounded
by grand-scale history, restored and preserved, maybe
shouldn't be deemed snobs.

When in Rome — this cliché has value for sure:
dwell and do as Romans. Lisette disjoined me from the
other hairstylists downstairs, maintaining a close eye on
my every move cutting clients upstairs beside Femme
Sistina's boutique lounge area. Stylists going out or
arriving strode past me and my clients, for days on end

refusing to acknowledge I existed. My partial ability to speak fluent Italian was the basic premise supporting an ineptitude attempting in-depth conversations with coworkers. Lisette, affixed as a famished mother hawk, translated whatever necessary dialogue between me and non-English-speaking clients. In an odd sense I felt chained, separated from staff below, similar to man-eating wild African animals held at bay beyond gladiators until slaughter's bloodshed hour. That is a frequent unfading impression, may've occurred two thousand years ago; but my imagination leans toward extravagance, revisiting Rome especially, in person or through memory. Not paying mind to others when they won't accept you isn't the end of anyone's world. Slowly but steadily my colleagues' presence had become comfortably translucent — only their noses visible, ever so slightly raised, strolling past the makeshift station Lisette created for me.

Down below, as in any busy salon, a stylist's personal working space usually starts out tidy of various equipment. All of a sudden around mid-morning, tools begin spilling outside drawers, cupboards, spreading wider across their countertops, exposing tangled cords, blow dryers, clippers, curling and flat irons, which lay about anywhere available — free from various combs, brush assortments, scissor collections, razors, not forgetting thinning shears, your hair's worst nightmare — with approximately one half dozen gooey, stench filled beauty products providing the international, artificial "finished look."

You're good, you know me by now, we're on the verge
of advantageous information, another product besides
a Mason Pearson brush, at least until 2015. In fifty
zillion beauty products available, two were among those
praiseworthy, whose ability to enhance hair exceeded
any sold. Were the other stylists working downstairs
so rude?— no, not really. They began each day opening
Femme Sistina's front door grumbling, "buongiorno";
although receptionist and retail clerk Loredana
was temporarily holding court, I assumed Lisette's
employees' 10 a.m. salutations included myself as
well. Lisette made her entrance about an hour after
everyone else. Later that day, nine hours lapsing, Femme
Sistina's charm-filled hostess carrying on several
conversations simultaneously in five languages, saw the
subterranean crew trudging by, individually mumbling
their dutiful "buonasera," leaving without pause —
again felt I was included.

I was consumed by skepticism about policies within
Lisette's salon, Rome too, perhaps Italy in general; she
continually (myself also under certain circumstance)
overstated through dramatization. Completely believing
her would've meant it was impossible by Italian law to
rid herself of an undesirable staff member, namely those
stylists barely sharing pleasantries, other than the aloof
(translated) "good morning" and "goodnight." Booted
not merely for the sake of being distant with her, but
everyone; clients too were without exception. Lisette's
beauty establishment, then pushing its four-decade span,

prospered by heavy tourist foot traffic, the reward of having such a stellar location.

After my second working trip, third to Rome, I eventually understood this wasn't just me exclusively toward whom Lisette's stylists displayed animosity. Their resentment was additionally directed at others who weren't Italians with lengthy lineage, recognized by Italian law— could've been Italy's ongoing unfavorable economy that soured them, I'm obviously speculating. According to Lisette an employee might commit a capital crime before their employer can legally dismiss them. Jobs in Italy come few and far between — once hired, employees apparently have the upper hand. Lisette's stylists, those individuals I encountered, epitomized a dysfunctional staff.

On the whole, throughout months spent there, here is my foremost complaint: many of those in Rome within the service industry unfairly lash out pent-up hostility, demonstrating aggressive behavior against others. This post beneath them, trembling with revulsion to think they should serve anyone, possibly with better lives elsewhere, rather than appreciate the reality of gainful employment. Capable existing true down below, maybe I, character *il diavolo*, shown distinct treatment by their employer — guest of honor, center stage, performing art as international window shoppers snooped by, fetching eight times Lisette's listed fee for haircuts. Me, perhaps the "Americano" stealing food from their family dinner table.

Lisette's senior male stylist might've begun working

downstairs when her physician husband, who since rests
at final peace, bought his young bride Femme Sistina
in 1958. Her deepest-rooted stylist at a place in life,
wearing glasses on the tip of his beak, argyle v-neck
sweater vest over gingham shirt, full Windsor-knotted
cravat, moderately coordinated pleated pants, and
orthopedic-style shoes, impeccable attire for an elderly
accountant's image. No way in hell could Lisette get him
out for good, although he'd snooze when he wasn't busy
skillfully making clients appear twenty years older than
they should've. Concluding drawn-out negotiations she
declined to pay him by lump sum what he demanded for
his early retirement, so there Giovanni stayed, standing
out like a sore thumb.

An era foregone, those beguiling years seemingly
vanished without a trace, as then Elizabeth Taylor or
Sophia Loren may very well have visited this aging stylist.
Giovanni, then a much younger man, shampooed, set,
and combed out those stars' hair, he undoubtedly created
swanky hairdos — pristine petals for Liz, Italian c-sides
on Sophia, Rome's leading lady — yet followed the trend
later using blow dryer, round roller brushes, and curling
iron. By my observation, his manipulating those tools
appeared as foreign by comparison to either of us holding
a spirited conversation in each other's mother tongue.

There I found something which saddened me: he'd
made accommodation for the modernized woman;
little did she realize what lost art form in which he was
a natural talent. If there were only one choice of stylist

I must report, this gentleman was the most somber —
hadn't ever seen a smile on his face. He'd come upstairs,
glasses typically hanging from a chain around his neck,
periodically stopping at Lisette's front desk to review
that day's receipts, putting them on for more perfect
vision. Maybe he forgot that particular afternoon to
remove those spectacles; stepping away before going
back downstairs, Giovanni picked up on his way and held
what had been my only after-cutting product, a crème
hairdressing — grinning broadly, said, "I remember
theese," pronouncing the Vitapointe tube "*veeta pont.*"

I didn't expect waving a tube of Vitapointe anywhere
here and there would've acted the Pied Piper, producing
one glorious Italian merriment procession through
their slender winding streets. Had I not been convinced
Vitapointe was the ideal crème for hair, Lisette's senior
stylist would've reconfirmed any doubt. Under the
impression he'd not spoken much English came surprise
upon hearing his eloquent speaking so with a patrician
Roman delivery. That discontinued 1.7-ounce tube broke
enough ice with him; whatever he said to the others
downstairs I'll not ever know, though each had warmed
up, saying goodbyes before closing their workday as every
night, though now, magically, all eyeballs glanced toward
my direction. While none became best of friends, they
were at last cordial from then on. In turn, our friendly
associations made Lisette discontent; as it happened, part
of her permitted my existence to place a wedge between
herself and those stylists she couldn't release, while hiring

Kobe beef for their coveted styling chairs remained this employer's ultimate goal.

Didn't take any effort to pack my gear: two cutting combs, a wide-tooth comb, pair of section clips, styling drape, travel-size water spray bottle, no brushes — can't properly sanitize the Mason Pearson brand for public use — one favored scissor, another as standby, and Vitapointe (pre-2015); whoosh I was gone. The drawback of staying that stripped down, having minimal equipment and limited product quantity, is I'm stranded if any items are misplaced or lost. Since 9/11 my shears prevent me from exclusive carry-on — this compact satchel must be checked as luggage. Strange, I hadn't any recollection leaving behind that tube of Vitapointe with Femme Sistina's senior stylist before departing Rome — blimey, finishing my next client in Manhattan felt somewhat incomplete without it.

✝

✢

Out Of The Kasbah

Should be common knowledge that tap water and its accompanying chemicals dry out the skin; hair isn't any exception. On days pressed for time, we'll either forget or, too hurried, forfeit an application of skin moisturizer after a shower — towel drying, getting dressed, and flying outdoors. This won't disable us, we'll pull through; if carried on indefinitely our skin's top layer will soon appear through repeated neglect completely flakey and gray, caused by dead skin.

Why we use moisturizer on skin is exactly the explanation for instance of argan oil's importance to hair. Even though I've suggested conditioning daily, the rinsing process eliminates most of what had been applied, further absorbing more natural sebaceous oil through towel drying.

A perfect morning scenario is coming out of the shower without tangles. Recall, conditioner was combed through while showering, smoothing any which were present; rinsing by the water's pressure had then left hair tangle-free. No reason to comb after drying off, thereby removing or rearranging its characteristic individual texture; also avoid wrapping your hair in a turban, mashing and retangling everything all over again.

After showering, gently blot hair using your bath sheet; grab then a smaller hand towel while changing — microfiber towels are better yet — drying in this same delicate scrunching manner. My advice for even distribution of plant-based oil onto hair: leave some dampness remaining.

A dose of plant-derived oil, both simple and tricky. It's every beauty after-product you'll ever need; although if you put a size larger than an average green pea or corn kernel speck onto the palm of your hand, you've probably poured out too much, more than what's necessary — half that amount on finer hair. 100% almond, coconut, argan, avocado or grapeseed oil is beyond compare, producing subtle effects you'll see and feel. Few other oils or imitations have such creamy consistency; others may not be as easy to regulate an application's amount.

Don't overfeed oil directly through hair — instead emulsify by rubbing it onto the palm of your hands first. I've suggested clients do precisely what pointers I'm giving you, and inquired upon their second appointment if they were able to locate some plant-derived oil online. "Yeah, but I didn't like it, my hair looked too greasy." Pouring a pea-size drop onto my hand I questioned, "Did you use about this amount?" "Oh no, forgot that part, I used way more than at drop."

Another misstep partial listeners don't catch, when I recommend they tip their head upside-down, saying, "Always apply from your nape toward the front area; done in this manner won't get its initial abundance around both temples and forehead's hairline, giving an appearance you desperately need a shampoo." While finer hair may without doubt require only half the normal proposed amount, curlier, thicker texture will easily absorb two, possibly three times that size, applied in separate portions, each spread through correctly, instead of accumulating a bunch throughout during one application.

Your intention isn't to go after an over-stylized "finished look" per se; plant-based oils are a hairdressing remedy from former years, leaving hair supple and radiant, not artificial.

One Vitapointe tube lasted for months and stayed approximately the price of a Ronald McDonald Happy Meal. How a beauty industry monster could have profited by selling Vitapointe is anybody's guess, other than sheer volume. How ironic could this be — after a multitude of years Vitapointe was discontinued, dare say their profit margin wasn't up to snuff. When another speck couldn't be squeezed from my last Vitapointe tube, I tried several suitable plant-based oils, and surprisingly switched without trouble — bet they're not going anywhere soon.

I'm thrilled you selected this book; other than clients pursuing their Jehrcuts, personal income for me at this juncture pauses there. Reiterating I'll vow on all

things hallowed, Jean included: Mr. Haute Coiffure has
no financial gain endorsing any beauty products listed
within these pages.

Two traditional, although quite different products —
firstly, your British allegiance, a Mason Pearson brush,
By Appointment to Her Majesty The Queen; another,
plant-derived oils, my gratis representation, hailing from
Queens, New York.

✝

✝

Bless Me Father

Possibly you have also faced a long-term challenge,
which after recurring themes went absolutely nowhere,
other than of course the headaches produced by
connected stress, eventually settling, "This is an
unworkable situation." Predicaments such as these
hadn't at that precise moment found most of us
tickled pink; afterward, following unabating tenacious
magnified investigation turning ourselves inside-out,
we reach an epiphany. Those of us, the slowpokes, don't
escape resisting change, we just aren't aware this already
happened before an unfamiliar concept impacted our
lives, having yet embraced it.

I manifested myself in 1991, by a jumbo gulp, into that
gut of an obscure heinous situation no person should
ever need to confront. Mercifully, in the fullness of time,
I convoked my vicious vexation to our duel, mine an
addict's existence which deteriorated over twenty years.
Mine were an overpowering propensity for refined drink
containing alcohol washing down smokeable herbs,

inhaling vapors and resins, assorted psychedelics, fungi, cactus, plus synthetic, polished off powders, uptown or downtown, interspersed with a galaxy of pills, all for me ingestible. I'd come to be my very own detestable beast who swallowed himself up.

And it was also said, dear brethren, that Jonah, devoured by a whale-type creature, found eventual light of day, spit out upon shore; I hope after suffering at such great lengths he might've discovered himself strewn across warmer Caribbean sands, not jagged rocks along the Bering Sea.

Ten years we'll suppose is a sufficient period of worldly penance; I, as well, supervening inner turmoil, through clearheaded years, rose above that pit contaminated by despair into the sundrenched, towering Manhattan Condé Nast offices, for an interview with *Allure* magazine. Prior to arriving, our agreed pitch gave me the impression of being palatable — Jehr, single-name hairstylist, charging a whopping $1000 per Jehrcut. My assigned journalista hadn't any idea what I'd been through that previous decade, she had but a pair of loosey-goosey facts; rushed in, urging me, "We need to be kind of quick." Apparently she'd been pressed on deadline for other stories — *The Devil Wears Prada*, in real life.

No matter how I score interest among media, their first, non-intellectually profound question seemingly could go on morning, noon and night: "Which celebrities do you cut, Jehr?" I've mellowed considerably with age, rather than sensing my ego be categorically ignored;

every competitive lying hairstylist spouts the same answer to this question: "Taylor, Gwyneth, Gwen" — not for me, no thank you. Anything's feasible — perhaps a dozen different hairstylists could have combed through the same three famed women, surely anything can find legitimacy. None, though, probably struck a pose alongside Taylor, Gwyneth, or Gwen. Each hadn't doted over those stars hours on end; fifteen hundred clicks and popping strobes later, photos sent into hanky-panky post-production, an image then eternally up for grabs — adopted by fibbing hairstylists worldwide. Your powers of reasoning must be the judge in this final analysis; can a familiar hairstylist without living proof assert their celebrity client list actually so?

For years Hollywood film studios have missed out; they've lost tremendous revenue not creating a magnificent brand, right on their studio lot — Paramount *Salon de Beauté*. Halting future fashion magazine inquiries regarding who's cutting or coloring whom comes as word is leaked — famous people don't actually patronize salons, discreet hairstylists under confidentiality agreements visit their homes.

Pure contemplation alone of what Miley's, Gaga's or Cameron's next look shall be occupies that interval between their last public image blitz. There are always exceptions to broad generalizations — here's a novel thought, what if VIPs didn't expect infinite comped luxury services and merchandise? Any nincompoop understands celebrity approval is worth their weight

in precious gemstones; famous people scarcely pay
for services, if at all, hardly ever using themselves what
they endorse.

Because big-name hairstylists spend endless hours
on a handful of red carpet clientele, some gather multi-
million dollar funding, formulating talc into aerosol
sprays, labeling it theirs, with crafty titling: "dry shampoo."
Heck, why not, parabens by the truckload: methyl, propyl,
butyl, ethyl, blending also petroleum jelly and synthetic
fragrance inside handy tubs, expanding those ineffectual
non-eco-friendly product lines. Hollywood film studios
along with record companies continue taking a safe
bet, understanding consumers purchase what they see
through advertising even though it's garbage, finish it up
to run back, buying whatever actors, actresses, and singers
supposedly use. During the interim it wouldn't be such
a smart idea to hold anyone's breath, waiting around
until celebrities appear in droves, supporting any green
revolution challenging the beauty industry.

While I write, as mentioned, Jeanette compiles
research and fact-checks material, in addition to
transferring my lined pages no eyes other than Jeanette's
could possibly comprehend onto computer. These are
pencil scribbles, its first improvised rough draft, round
two proofreading I'll scribble over that, editing then a
third scribbling go-around. My manuscripts' initial handwritten muddled up sentences resemble Blackbeard's
treasure map; disarrayed pages comprising each book
demand angelic patience decoding before reaching

Jeanette's computer, her distance having composure
usually surpassing mine.

Whether she realizes or not, I couldn't be certain,
Jeanette frequently comments about vaguely related
material which steers writing's course. An unspecified
day later, through Jeanette's insight, I will notice
myself filling other pages which brought guiding light
into a subject her research unveiled. Recently Jeanette
mentioned studies at Stanford had indeed proven under
clinical test trials that young women, specifically their
self-image, are adversely affected by the beauty machine.
I'm not positive Mr. Haute Coiffure should entirely
modify midstream, referring to the beauty business
or industry being machine-like; however, that does
resonate prompts for major belated change. Before Avon
or LVMH executives get huffy in a tizzy, sensing their
contracts be prematurely terminated, not another worry
— this revolution, unlike Marie Antoinette's, won't
permit actual severing of heads. Clever money-grubbers
as they are will over time unquestionably concoct
completely different lines of product, marketing "inner"
beauty — in fact, it's already well underway, the Dove
Campaign for Real Beauty.

We invariably discover certain celebrities becoming
pigeonholed into parodies of their onscreen characters,
a mold troublesome to break from. Few great stars
expand their career, those who evolved using celebrity
for higher significance, the humanitarians, a sincere
Audrey Hepburn did, today Bono. Campaigning,

through public relation motives toward popular trend, as example, fundraising for that most recent global disaster, a disingenuous quality broadly viewed, making evident some well-known faces care about what the majority empathizes, if this exposure rebuilds their fainted limelight, while also handsomely translating marked deductions April 15th.

How, without target, I stay attracted toward proclivity favoring innovative culture is unclear — why, at least for myself, neither here nor there. Held firm early, inadvertently cutting celebrities before their established notoriety. What groundbreaking trend, styling punk rock bands in 1977 — today, status quo, seen throughout shopping malls across most every continent. Came to terms with my appetite for an existence at the cusp, opposing those hungry, yet both unoriginal and idle — arriving after their prey had been taken down by Mr. Haute Coiffure, one ambitious predator.

✝

✝

AUTHENTICITY COMPROMISED

I met a young African American woman in cosmetology
school; we began attending freshman class on the same
day with an eclectic motley mix, equally diverse as us.
Caryn struggled as a new mother, no husband nor steady
mate; she planned to bridge Welfare into income styling
hair, before, quoting her, "making it big someday." Passing
her workstation months later, I heard a raspy, lower-key
monotone voice, with recently-transplanted New York
accent murmuring, "c'mere, ya busy?— do sum'n for me,
hold the stencil over here above my ear, I wanna bleach
this star there." She cut out from cardboard, covering
with aluminum foil her individual stamp, stenciling
on closely cropped hair a usual five-point insignia. An
alteration I've considered colossal, from Caryn Johnson
to six-pointed Jewish star Whoopi Goldberg, Caryn's
recognized trademark.

Anybody else who spent just under one year with
Caryn Johnson wouldn't have ever guessed in seventy
billion years what she resisted like some bubonic plague:

coming to be the woman of color's morning edition,
for, let's face it, America's predominately white beauty
machine. For years they'd been dreads, then again not,
shaped meticulously blunt by a graduated neckline.
Depending what mood Whoopi's feeling, bluish hue
contact lenses today, green tomorrow, wardrobe matchy-
match synchronized with her *View* co-hosts five mornings
every week. Caryn Johnson wouldn't have exchanged two
words with any Barbara Walters type in 1976, other than
possibly "hey" and a definite "later," probably mocking
her after walking away; we'd read Caryn's lips pouring
one vulgar stream of sarcasm.

Having banked millions, plus loads of personal
caricature, most, such as Whoopi, with a platform simply
don't trigger positive influence in others. Is it they lack
social responsibility? Perhaps the entertainment and
beauty industry — machine, if you prefer — censors
conscience, threatening their Wonder Bread and
margarine, a poor substitute on anybody's payday, living
or tombstone's epitaph, especially those with sway. Much
as I've found myself drawn to privilege allocated by
deal making, the end-all result seemed flat; endorsing
any number of beauty companies' inferior product lines
hadn't substance. I imagine I'll reflect, as most do in
years ahead, currently wishing what I've aspired to will
be contagious, hopefully noticing lives were improved by
Mr. Haute Coiffure's proposals.

At some point we'd suspect particular famous
personalities are so enormously solvent, they'd not stoop

to accept lesser quality parts for another seven-figure check — Robert De Niro, Dustin Hoffman. (Why unfairly isolate Whoopi?) How could Hoffman or De Niro add the *Fockers* series to an otherwise near-spotless body of work, rather than enjoy their previous success? Smarmy Ben Stiller's an entirely different circumstance altogether. Had the ongoing Malibu-Tribeca, bicoastal private jet-setting rates driven our beloved Ratso Rizzo and Travis Bickle into transparent glory?

✝

VAINGLORIOUS

Did Bernie Madoff defraud those remarkable entertainers;
hadn't they any other recourse? Now then, let's give, for
instance, Barbra Streisand her due benefit of the doubt —
say she was cash strapped and in truthfulness desperately
needing not one but two *Fockers* appearances to cover
delinquent bills; maybe not Madoff, but another crooked
financier, bilking Streisand's fortune bone dry.

Obviously Barbra hadn't wisely elected to choose
the higher road, while others into their seventies,
ordinary folks, naturally gravitate toward a richness of
one's soul, those immersed in delivering humanistic
assets, which peers seem inspired by; additionally, an
abnormal upstanding role model for society's younger,
impressionable members.

Using Streisand, for example, as the positive
emulation fans this entire world might look up to,
isn't very accurate, considering Barbra carved out and
paved before her any formidable diva's pampered path.
Spoiled rotten to the core does not necessarily have

eternity written on it. For whatever rationale, Streisand, out of every imaginable hairstyle money could afford, yearns to wear these last fifty years her blown out, flat-ironed bob with highlights. Had Jon Peters created that blasé signature look for her?— he progressed, kudos to him.

I don't foresee any situation in our near or distant future of Barbra Streisand becoming spokesperson for the American Red Cross. I'm not talking about a twenty-second spot between Morgan Freeman and Jane Fonda either, for whatever dreadful event hasn't hit yet. She'd urgently require a believable appearance; Streisand couldn't wear the bob she has. Shall we have her take a steamy hot shower; soak away the snooty feeling of superiority; shampoo, condition, towel dry; sitting still, without saying anything while Mr. Haute Coiffure performs his artistry?

Bothersome eyesore, protruding my styling cape on her lap; send we must for a manicurist — her squared off French manicure reeks archaic ostentation. Please ask Barbra's manicurist to pack lightly — polish remover, cotton balls, nail clipper; have those silk-wrapped stumped ends trimmed eighty percent, filing with her finger's contour, cuticle nippers for strays, followed by suede buffer and vitamin E oil. We can work around the manicurist simultaneously — no problem, switching sides our professionalisms' *pas de deux*. Combing from Barbra's ends toward her scalp, observe, listening to what the hair's exactitude tells us.

"Oh thank El Shaddai, you finally sat this woman down; she hasn't listened to us since who knows when. We're choking to death wrapped inside those aluminum foils every six weeks. Why she insists on beige highlights, when our gray is in every way unimpeded by impurities and contaminants, it's absolutely beyond us. Mr. Haute Coiffure what would you do about those awful sticky hair products she applies right after shampooing and conditioning?— we don't ever sense actually being clean. How long do you think it would take until our elasticity returns back to normal?— it's like a torture rack being stretched every day. You know anything about these burns covering us; she keeps purchasing blow dryers and flat irons hotter than the previous ones. Who are you, Mr. Haute Coiffure, is your identity a passing episode? Will we be released from Barbra Streisand's tyranny, then someday yield to her abuse again? Why won't she accept our intrinsic worth?"

As if to till a garden's soil, ever so confidently massaging Barbra's shoulders using both reassuring hands, hers this delicate flower's dominium, she adore forever upcoming beauty by inceptive preparation. Streisand resists confrontation; her trust beckoned from the muscle tissue's surrender, signaling to Mr. Haute Coiffure she's submitted; his calming hand's pressure gradually releases, holding tools momentarily, they willingly rescue persecution's witness.

Any prospect Streisand hold her lips closed while Mr. Haute Coiffure listens to Barbra's hair, permitting omakase, is about the plausibility of Hollywood spearheading an uprising from its Beverly Hills mutilation mecca, à là Donnatella Versace — becoming instead a warm-hearted rendition, growing beautiful as Jamie Lee Curtis and Daniel Day-Lewis.

An across-the-board grumble I'm sure you've heard, as I, starting conversation with clients, often open dialogue inquiring, "Have you seen any good movies lately?" Practically every client I've asked that question during the past twenty years has given me this response, "There hasn't been much out I have any interest in seeing." Another entirely separate issue frequently surfaces — prices at the box office; but, this isn't by any means their main deterrent, hooray streaming movies. Those studio executives carrying out authority, what scripts should be produced onto film, apparently haven't the foggiest notion what their audience is about. Jaded Tinseltown, an understatement; imposing yachts, private jets, multiple luxury automobiles, Iron Chef-prepared meals inside their mansions' gourmet kitchens, none uncommon.

BY JEHR SCHIAVO
WRITING AS GERARD SAINT D'ANGELO

✟

WE ARE DIVINE

An extended period in certain parts of LA could lead many
to contemplate severe modifications, myself included.

"Jeanette, do I look fat to you? See that guy over there,
the one wearing all white, we're probably close in age,
who looks older, me or him? Do I have more wrinkles
or does he? Think I should grow my hair out a half inch,
bleach it, hide any gray, visit the tanning salon until I'm
Cabo brown?"

What Jeanette doesn't ever tell me: "Yeah Jehr,
go right ahead, lose fifteen or twenty pounds, switch
from wearing all black into white exclusively, have your
face lifted two inches; while you're there, get some chest
implants, a butt lift wouldn't be so bad either, become
blonde, spray yourself terra-cotta, we'll catch the next
flight to Acapulco, you'll enter their local cliff-diving
contest, maybe splitting that dense skull might return any
former ability of sound reasoning you've ever
had before spending time on Rodeo Drive back where
it belongs."

Jeanette barely says anything that snide to me when I pose similar trivial questions; ours is deep affection the lucky share. She'll glance over at that tan, chiseled guy, twenty-five years younger, dressed wearing all-white, slouched against his silver Maybach, smart device one hand, brown tortoiseshell Persol shades the other, bolstering my deflated ego fabricating fiction, "You look much better than him." Believe it or not, that's the way authenticity rolls, falsification under imperfect situations; Mr. Haute Coiffure, too, faces his insecurities.

A sane person mustn't disagree, shouting slanderous remarks, "Mr. Haute Coiffure, the conspiracist — his ideology is unfounded, he's biased against the beauty industry he lambastes, don't read another word."

Alright, fine, nobody's pointing a pistol against anybody's brain, no one is forced into reading anything; see for yourself, on front covers at newsstands anywhere. Don't know where to begin — start with O magazine. Mr. Haute Coiffure should put up a to-do. For over thirty years Winfrey delivers her billionaire-next-door distorted message. Shouldn't we empower being true to ourselves first, before preaching all across America? Whatever allegedly improves lives, Oprah's all over it, like white on rice. Have for yourself a suitable gander at the covers of her magazine. There's an enormous difference between Jeanette telling me a little white lie and Oprah permitting relentless images of herself, that the imposter. Her O magazine covers are complete and pure malarkey, conveying false expectations directed toward women, tens of millions, whom she swears up and down to genuinely help. Ready to board your Gulfstream G650, Oprah? That private weight clinic in Bhutan starts at eight p.m. Pacific Standard Time, maybe Emeril wouldn't mind whipping some snacks together during your flight.

Talk about high chances of blacklisting myself; if that were the case, this I christen, Mr. Haute Coiffure's OWN kiss of death. No book of the month club through Oprah's rubber stamping, not in this lifetime, given her topical disposition. LA producers, what probability, sending this or future manuscripts to their offices, becoming licensed film rights anytime soon? It's okay, me and Mr. Haute Coiffure are not pliable pieces of clay.

Have you said to yourself, "Jehr does have quite the unorthodox communiqué, but what should I do about it?"

It would be the senseless argument to fight our government, a different plot — those Washington D.C. characters are much more foreboding than 90210. This whole country's population, fifty uniting states, wouldn't ever consider banding together to alter the Internal Revenue Service's unjustifiable, astronomical penalty and interest fees, if every taxpayer defiantly went on strike. "That's it, I'm completely disgusted, no one else is paying their taxes, neither will I." These protests and strikes occur frequently in the private sector; customers join together boycotting particular corporations; if it were an oil company, within days prices would drastically dip at gas pumps everywhere.

I've a triple-prong pitchfork, with heroic outlaw attitude. Here's your visual exercise: construct a bonfire, large as it could ever ignite, this one shall be prodigious; our power source, though, isn't wood — ours is that toxic combination which often causes mushroom blowups, similar to epic firestorms watched across action movie screens. No matter how profitable a relationship theirs is, bonded as conjoined twins, that deep-seated connection, aesthetics represented through an iron-willed entertainment and beauty industry continues presenting life-size Barbie dolls in the flesh — Sofía Vergara, Jennifer Aniston, Beyoncé. Their incestuous link having squeaking gears démodé; here or somewhere symbolically, torch this interdependence up into a Herculean smoke plume, followed by its heap of vivid flames. One could say righteous adaption often rises from ashes, having proprietary right initiating an impassioned advanced sense of inner beauty.

Heartbroken, I'm recently reminded, how can we possibly proceed any longer without another two hours of Joan Rivers kibitzing what celebrities wore who, each spring modeling their way into Hollywood Boulevard's Dolby Theatre before hopefuls receive those golden Oscars? Nobody said take the Academy Awards away. Down to business, there's no doubt in my mind excellence on screen would return again, having memorable modern film noir potential, after dissolving the two-headed machine feeding each other, impairing trusting bystanders. Cary Grant didn't choose plastic

surgery; neither did Alfred Hitchcock nor Grace Kelly —
acclaimed trio those three, presented their timeless gift
to us, classic movies we'll certainly revisit.

Not my favorite top pick for preferred rock 'n' roll
band, though I stay enormously fond of Metallica's
present-day milk and honey life. Theirs also was a story
concerning an inferno, started by refusing the traditional
music industry route — instead they sold Metallica
records out of their car after gigs touring for beer money.
I admire such unmitigated defiance which ultimately
brought Elektra Records down on their knees, signing
Metallica's unheard-of advances — couch surfing to
platinum album-lined walls. Their outspoken drummer's
cash-purchased former Tiburon estate garnered three
hundred sixty degree views of San Francisco's bridges,
bay and islands dotting her, safeguarding too his museum
quality art collection. What, no hair plugs, fake tan, nor
plastic surgery, Lars?

I've observed the cycle in fashion change, 2016 on its
fourth rotation since 1976; all inbound roads directed
themselves to a central point of inspiration, rock 'n' roll.
The day I see Patti Smith consistently color her hair,
maybe Neil Young purchasing his toupée or Iggy Pop
surgically stretching those hard-earned facial wrinkles,
anyone who'd wish should then boast, "I told you all
along, hot air, full of conspiracy theory that Mr. Haute
Coiffure — he's such a card."

✝

✦

INSIDE OUT

He who rats out on his own profession — doesn't this
person have intention knowingly in advance? Yes, in all
conceivability, premeditated for Frank Serpico; but he
couldn't have possibly foreseen such a degree of success
coming down the pike before uncovering New York City's
Police Department's flagrant corruption. Sooner or later,
for those donning a rare twenty-four hour conscience, it
begins to weigh heavy; what was morally right outweighed
Frank's badge's unjust normalcy. They too, both Karen
Silkwood and Erin Brockovich — neither held up their
white flags under pressure, no need acquiescing to fear.
Women, perhaps more so, desire pertinent charge toward
greater balance, improving lower standards from present
male dominance, a destructive masculine path oppressing
quality in life of others. Not a woman nor man pursuing
fairness achieves their platform alone; courage must also
give pivotal credit where credit's deserved.

    After providing an outline, suitably done, compiling
sufficient information, authors of either sex may and

then again might not receive earned publishment. Equally important to this writer's content, their prospective literary agent, who immediately requires without any exception his or her concise reply upon hearing, "Does anyone follow you — what is your platform?"

Lacking serious media attention, more or less, in any socially responsible rat's case, would be their crucifixion; missing an ever-so-important resurrection, dime a dozen, next number to the counter. Remaining crucial, that key of incalculable worth, media professionals who enlighten humanity's awareness. Recognition of the newshound has been taken for granted, unfair, yet acceptable, despite breaking seminal stories, their identities go forgotten. "What was that person's name at the *New York Times* who broke Serpico's story?" Thankless careers, depending of course on how enlarged their self-image was. Is it adequate that any press individual later say if ever asked, "Yes that's right, Brockovich was my story, I was first to profile Erin, you're quite welcome." It seems as though by a certain stage this overlooked reporter could become callous delivering breaking news, unless their story is significant, bringing widespread attention to an article with the controversy of Karen Silkwood's. That groundbreaking piece furnished this now-established writer's ongoing comfort — maybe a second property, Amagansett or Palm Springs, hanging their hat so to speak, wool night watch cap on frigid winter evenings, her summer afternoon shade provided by floppy chapeau, mixed with his baseball hats in between.

The scattered remaining literary agents shouldn't have anything to whine about. Doesn't make any difference whatsoever if their writer finishes a Homeric novel or mine, piercing its gaping nonfiction wound straight into the beauty industry machine's underbelly; they'll get twenty percent regardless. Means of the world function exquisitely in closed-door meetings; what we don't acknowledge surely won't offend us. Did Silkwood, Brockovich, or Serpico make preferential agreed arrangements with their media entrée?— rather dubious behavior for any one of those three, highly unethical also; press members as a rule abide by stringent, common moral code. To accomplish a published manuscript traditionally or not obtain its publishing, this, the writer's eighty-percent inquiry. Pit bull mentality concerning ill-guided beauty, in general, are not the primary whys and wherefores of some grandiose exposé, especially within fashion related magazines, where wide-eyed subscribers stand as that journal's captivated audience.

Those bold enough to pare away layer after layers sooner or later reach the crux. Among a vast array of clientele, no single beauty treatment they obtained elsewhere fulfilled the client's inner gratified unspoken voice, having unvarnished endurance. Innumerable services received by many contributed to continued emptiness. She will sit before mirror, presuming her exterior's reflection were overhauled by various forms of FDA-approved chemicals, giving at best a temporary sense of newness — danger came, however, no warning

included. While a hairstylist paints color onto foil
squares, weeks after applying her keratin treatment —
an esthetician's biting chemical peel shortly thereafter
— tomorrow gel manicure, pedicure in-progress, or the
pre-op felt pen guiding that plastic surgeon's master plan
next week, will this client and patient finally contemplate
self-content? If her hair is straight enough, having
ample blonde highlights, face satisfactorily smooth,
gel manicure, pedicure adequately pleasing Kathie Lee
Gifford, lips Angelina Jolied — had frequenting the
medical day spa reached an internal void, or might those
visits only hold hostage what anguish she perchance
walked inside with, still increasing and unanswered?

People will hand bosses every kind of alibi — they
have a doctor or dentist appointment, parent-teacher
conference, any old tired excuse for their fix-me-quick
beauty hour. They enjoyed their hot stone massage,
shampoo, or thirty-minute conditioning treatment; had
these services, though, touched life's elusive inner beauty
tranquility? Once genuinely apprehended, hers or his
indelibly lives on.

Maestro Richard Avedon, dramatic portraitist
dissimilar to any other; within each face bearing aged
weathered lines, unfurrowed, possibly furrowed brow,
mouth at ease or strained — beyond every facial feature,
his subject's eyes express the heart's revelation.

Having personal encounters catching glimpses
into my patrons' psyche, through time I'll gather their
trust, hearing, "My mother died when I was five." The

yoga devotee, herself quote-unquote an energy healer, occasionally mentioned not understanding why she's so compelled to take care of everyone around her, though appointment after appointments persists in verbal abuse toward those she loves behind their backs. A personality split, divided in half, two different separate parts, nurturer and spiteful grouch. Oblivious, not recognizing why she has the inclination to be everyone's mother, while preserving resentment having tremendous loss at such an early age.

I listen intently, hearing lengthy confidential conversations about my clients' abuses and abusings. Mental, infrequent but not out of the question, sexual complications, and also physical dilemma, obesity, anorexia, bulimia, those addicted to compulsion, including visits into their psychotherapist's office twice weekly. Perhaps human nature, a continuous scheduling of burdensome beauty appointments, seeking top-level hair colorist, cutter, manicurist, masseuse, esthetician, plastic surgeon, followed up purchasing shopping bags stuffed with unnecessary associated recommendations — however, still nothing sustainable — only on fleeting occasion was serenity temporarily captured.

Typical salon acoustics can't block out nearby jabbering. "My husband just dumped me for a man." "Girl, I've been telling you all along he was twisted, should have listened to me, sweetie." Beauty salons forever and a day not only breed superficial services, but also motor mouth gossip, neither exactly promotes inner beauty — can it? Until declaring an offensive attack, crusading with diligence to claim victory over this beauty industry adversary, which began encroaching women's psyches mid-twentieth century when most drank the Kool-Aid, it shall remain socially acceptable.

No blow out, flat iron, hair color, highlights, lowlights, extensions, straightening treatments, permanent waves, acrylic nail preference, dermal fillers nor tummy tuck will bring resolution to neglected personal issues of depth. A bankrupt journey, seeking uninterrupted beauty everywhere, except the single place which counts most.

✝

✝

HOODOO ON THE BAYOU

How Mr. Haute Coiffure discovered himself scheduling
New Orleans' sauciest, an entertaining saga, but too
involved; anyway, if a brief explanation were possible
this could come off as bragging — alright, you twisted
my arm, it stemmed from working in Rome, happy
now? Be that as it may I engaged myself every two
months reserving an executive hotel suite outside the
French Quarter, maintaining cuts for a hysterically
polite collection of persons with bizarre dispositions.
Treacherous bunch —they knew each other for ages,
years before their children went to school together, those
kids now starting families themselves. They'd often arrive
early for appointments while I was still cutting, both
women overtly complimenting one another, sounding
perfectly delightful, dense, upper crust, Southern
chitchat. Minutes after my previous client delivered
a fifteen-minute praline-coated goodbye to the next
intrusive appointment, arriving early expecting dish, I
heard her hungry earful, smack talking who'd just left, not

skipping any remarks about those family and friends soon on their way over.

In light of those women being skilled manipulators through conversation dripping with Louisiana etiquette, prying information from an outfoxed best friend, Mr. Haute Coiffure also delved, having intentions to manipulate, but with positive purpose. Describing negatively the appearance of a former patron here shouldn't be misunderstood.

"How could he speak so ruthlessly — when she reads what he's written about her here, she'll feel absolutely crushed."

Nah, folks have rugged skin down there in the Big Easy. In order to case study further, investigating my hypothesis, after explaining myself upside down and sideways, I took another direction, making a clear choice, throw currency at them.

Her husband appeared every bit the part of a reliable pediatrician approaching retirement as he could ever present himself. His wife was the target of my scheming technique, which I've too at times imposed upon other clients elsewhere, because its outcome brought complete recovery from that particular person's garish style. Cosmetics can draw a Tammy Faye Bakker unappealing quality — clumpy mascara, foundation caked-on-troweled-over, paste-like harlequin rouge and clown lipstick; my patron's grandchildren became accustomed — other kids meanwhile, like it or not, stunned with fright.

Several appointments later cutting this woman, I found for my taste unsatisfactory results. Discreetly prodding her into a more fashionable non-Fellini mode, bells went off in my head, *put your money where your mouth is.* Had I not known this woman, it would've been stupid silly offering her financial bait. This was really cunning of me to suggest bribery, "I'll pay you, if you'd stop coloring your hair." She wouldn't have ever taken my money, but I thought if there's any language this N'awlins gal understood, it was cold hard cash.

She was blushing through her pancake makeup when I about nearly begged on bended knees, "Switching to your natural silver-white hair from this blue-black will leave you an appearance looking fifteen years younger."

"I'm not sa sure Zjehr; I've been this culla evuh since I can rememba, what would friends think, don't ever mention this to muh huzbun."

Responding, "He has silver hair, works beautifully for him; he's as distinguished a person there is."

"Oh, I don't know; I'll have ta give it some thought now."

"Okay, but when I come back to town in eight weeks, if you haven't had it retouched, your regrowth should be at least an inch-and-a-half long, including what's grown out this far. If you don't see the colorist between now and then, your next appointment's on me."

Communicating by email with Jeanette after we left New Orleans, my client wrote she hadn't been to her hair colorist during the interim, but wasn't positive about having a change of heart, getting it colored before our upcoming scheduled visit.

Jeanette doesn't approve of my steering clientele by that method. Jeanette's pragmatic, especially with regards to our expenses; she doesn't appreciate paying for airfare and hotel accommodations, while putting "our" money where my mouth is. Mr. Haute Coiffure isn't a philanthropist privately funding inner beauty; Jeanette stands correct, my theory is mine. Patrons, if you please, you'll need to be responsible for yourselves, famiglia di Schiavo's economic matters mustn't become a liability by reason of client insecurity, sublimely sensible Jeanette's propriety.

I should make myself clear if anybody were curious — no, it wasn't pleasant visiting New Orleans after Hurricane Katrina. What had previously seemed like half the city wearing permanent smiles disappeared those next couple of years, leaving behind many desperately trying on happier faces for another resigned day. I realized business there would be coming to an end; yet my word was given — whether she'd act on receiving a complimentary cut was her prerogative.

My client could barely say hello, she was so excited. "Um gunna do it, muh huzbun's up fuh seeing my gray, friends are dyin' ta see what I look like when we're done. You're not gunna go make'n it too short are ya now Zjehr, I can't be getting all this dark stuff cut, we're doin' part taday, the rest when ya'll come back in seven or eight weeks, right?"

She settled it for me, if I wasn't so sure which month was to be our final there, that visit wouldn't have been exactly fair, leaving her as a work-in-progress.

Cutting over a king-size starched sheet pinned to my hotel room's carpet, her seated on the Metairie Courtyard Marriott's borrowed banquet chair, me, comb, scissors, no mirror in sight, not too surprising, she had already experienced letting go, after giving blessings for previous Jehrcuts.

"Um sa nervous Zjehr, ya sure we're doing the right thang; there's a whole lotta black hair comin' off, I'd rather not hurry ya now, but I just can't wait ta see."

Champagne bubbles she turned into, as though I popped a Dom Pérignon cork by that initial length of blue-black falling onto the white sheet below. Giddy and loopy, she couldn't much stay peaceful, any more than kids exiting Anaheim's busiest off-ramp.

Come to think of it, in a way this style appearing before my eyes cutting her hair blossomed into an updated, Tim Burton-revised Cruella de Vil. It takes greater artistic effort than I usually have within an hour to stay thoroughly satisfied one thousand percent — confines of the perfectionist — hers, though, were memorable and strikingly beautiful. By sliding my scissor blades toward her hairs' ends, I altered its former dowdy texture, becoming a halo of silver regrowth underneath, with exception — the very outer tips remaining an ominous blue-black aura, those garish and dastardly turned into wispy feather softness.

Postulate whatever you wish, an inch-and-a-half
of pure white blizzard, snow drift regrowth, enhanced
with a bitchin' blue-black smidgen still surviving isn't at
all common, it's drop-dead punk rock gorgeous — Demi
Moore, Catherine Zeta-Jones, Seth MacFarlane, by
diplomacy, have been advised. Proof is in the pudding's
final judge, my patron, not Mr. Haute Coiffure; even
if she might be walking out without paying — deal's
a deal. Reactions undergo every imaginable facial
expression, clients don't necessarily need to utter
anything. This variety of salty water her eyes welled
over with hadn't surged from sorrow; eventually gazing
in the mirror, hers were tears obviously dissimilar. Both
hands covered her mouth, it was wide open, she was
having a flabbergasted moment.

After catching her breath from shock, "Oh muh gawd,
I don't know what ta say, I feel sa diffrint Zjehr. Ya know
Um gunna pay ya fuh this, I don't care whut ya'll say.
Think it'd be too short if we cut off all the culla taday? I
mean it's kinda fun n'all see'n those lil'biddy black ends
fuh right now. Whuda y'all think, Jinett, ya like it?"

My patron's emotions said everything, she questioned
us, urgently wanting positive affirmation — should
go without saying, being genuinely fussed over after
transformation is part of the fee, that's a given. How a
woman can suddenly look fifteen pounds lighter, at least
that in years, significantly more attractive by apparent
joy alone, materialized metamorphosis with her newly
uncovered personal beauty's ownership. No junction

elsewhere during her previous three decades scheduling color appointments — I'll presume hers wasn't the same hairstylist for thirty years, although quite possibly could've been, yet didn't do what he or she should have done — long before Katrina or Mr. Haute Coiffure ever landed in New Orleans, had any of them been honest and frank with my client.

When we returned to the Metairie Courtyard eight weeks later, stylin' Cruella walked with calm leaving our suite, once camouflaged by artificial color, now washed clean having a quietude of knowingness, an unbelievable departure from the scatty, frazzled, animated character she no longer personified.

What I'm about to spill should through due course receive Jeanette's tolerance, but in the short run, I hear her micro avarice opinion she holds way down inside, reprimanding me, "What are you writing that for, why doesn't your Mr. Haute Coiffure partner learn some self-restraint, disciplining himself every now and then?"

If I weren't Mr. Haute Coiffure — I'd spend two-and-a-half hours coloring my client's hair, trimming her split ends, blow drying, ironing, then spraying it. Would this client be blissed out as Cruella? Tearing up, leaving thirty percent gratuity, planting coral lipstick marks on my cheeks; or as the young novice, another lifetime ago, listened to an insincere, "Love ya baby, call me, we'll go have drinks." I haven't swilled cocktails in twenty-six years, surely wouldn't be losing out on anything much without those party girls. Anyway, regarding

high-maintenance women, I hadn't ever felt mentally
connected there beyond two seconds. I'm always pleased
receiving thirty percent gratuity; however, what produces
the most pride is a sincere positive emotional response
by my patrons observing their mirrored reflections after
cutting, understanding life from that point forward
changed for betterment, mine included.

Who, I'll ask, Jeanette or me, would grow more
nauseated observing Mademoiselle Barbie weeping in
reference to how beautiful she perceived herself, by the
last spritz of designer volumizing spray? Mademoiselle
Barbie hadn't any interest living another path but hers,
puddle-sized. Some seize behavior attaining native acuity
when they're young, others older, less aware, continue
life regressing. Not many exist entirely unscathed by the
past, feeling choked up, coming to know all that hooey
invested desiring beauty brought on as years wouldn't
wait nor hide, theirs too were a variation of garish
and dastardly resemblance which could've easily been
avoided, like Lady de Vil.

Did stylin' Cruella, if truth be told, actually require
an inspired Jehrcut bringing her a sense of elegance?
In the event Jeanette permits that immediate previous
sentence passage, Mr. Haute Coiffure plans on officially
naming my amore *Générale d'Armée*, triumphantly leading
women who've had it up to here away from their obsolete
beauty regimens, oppressed by preconceived notions,
obstructing illumination of beauty's inner source.

✝

✝

CROWNING SILHOUETTE

A flock in flight formation, methodical unison, creating their future guiding movement — however rapid, whichever direction, whatever distance, wherever powered — together, they too as individuals must soar into the unknown.

We first commit a dipping swipe of our toes before diving into an unfamiliar swimming pool, it's natural. Nobody, I believe, would jump right in — we'll examine those waters instinctually. Don't let hair toy with you. Only when in your liking, comb all of it away from your face — this is that genuine article, the real McCoy work of art. Recently cleansed and moisturized, your facial features are the essential factor. Studying ourselves may seem daunting, but you mustn't concern yourself; most exercises we haven't tried before will frequently meet awkwardness.

At a place and time making exception before mirror during consultation I'll hold my exacting client's hair back; we'll peer together into her face assisted by the mirror's reflection. Ever so close, fractions within a centimeter, not using contact with my fingertips, I follow the outline of each cheekbone, then jawline, onto her chin — there's no chicanery from me.

Some other hairstyling sorcerer motions upward toward inquisitive eyes, the method David Copperfield uses, fluttering his monarch butterfly fingers, enticing that client's enchantment, merely supporting morale by mysterious sleight of hand.

No one is obligated to me — live in a dream world, choose whomever moves you, allow that imaginary person to draw your structural perfection, bringing into vision an arresting facial quality.

Heat, an Andy Warhol reference, 1982 until 1984, was my first solo endeavor; *Schiavo*, the second of two galleries, boomed through 1989 — a different location, still thoroughly intermingled art and beauty. I operated each business functioning with dual purpose — at the second of these addresses, a spartan loft space, others were by my side also styling hair. Over this eighty-four-month period at combined locations, I held one-person art exhibitions, not once hanging any group shows, other than San Francisco's Presidio Hill School's fundraiser consisting of first, second, and runner-up winners from a student body competition, spanning adorable kindergarteners to pugnacious eighth-graders. Other, serious gallery owners curate a single artist's work every month, sending invitations for open bar soirées; I lacked Larry Gagosian's dedication. Travel for hair-related ambition is one cause I'll vindicate subtracting fourteen months of seven years, give or take another half-dozen rebalancing from a solid month submerged into an exhibitor's psychosis — common in those creating profound work, the artist must exist unruffled, that gallery owner's unwritten responsibility.

Whether in my galleries, another's, or museums exhibiting modern work, frames for the most part are absent. Looking back upon pieces of art I've appreciated, including the Impressionist floor at Musée D'Orsay, I can't recollect specific frames, only that magnum opus within. Artists throughout bang-up periods — Michelangelo, Rembrandt, Renoir — no world-class curator would deliberate presenting those master exhibitions unframed. Modern art, on the other hand, put forth in such stylistic frameworks are obviously centuries past this once-status quo.

Current observation of present-day paintings: a stretched canvas, edges revealing nonchalant rawness, drips and splatters, paint unsystematically affixed, hurried, not wanting one speck incomplete, or time ran out, the artist simply leaving their studio with work unfinished.

Up in a villainous 1980s Gramercy Park penthouse — visiting ML, trashing ourselves senselessly, customary then to any evening's outing which inevitably slammed into the following morning's daybreak, both still annihilating our systems — there, in her abode, I viewed an imposing series of Chagalls hanging above my former accomplice's sofa. I'd seen tons of refined art stoned, although hers I could report absolutely nothing about. All, probably close to seven, were interchangeably

framed, the entire grouping gold, gaudy, ornate, new
money overdone — her drug smuggler roommate's fault.
Having no memory what Marc Chagall himself expressed
on canvas, for me arrived displaying art so elaborately,
an era I personally don't welcome with open arms,
self-debauched or not.

A few hundred years ago in history, perhaps this pansy
powdering the King and Queen's wigs, ensconced by their
palace's extraordinary framed artwork, couldn't resist
thinking to himself, "I am also an artiste," embellishing
royal patrons, as that nameless framer had selected for
Vermeer. Accessorizing seventeenth- or eighteenth-
century regal attire surely required endless yards of fabric,
much more than our clothing today; their wardrobe
demanded Italian wedding cake-proportion hair, right up
the alley for her majesty's gown to an afternoon tea jam
session amid violin, flute, cello, and harpsichord.

Fashion evolved — female billionaires nowadays
actually dress and transport themselves from boudoir to
sprawling dining hall without a Queen's bevy of assistants
escorting this modern, affluent woman. Meanwhile
elsewhere, at some well-off woman's preeminent London
salon, had it been circa Sassoon, right until this very
trendsetting minute, that benchmark of envy, where
hairstylists the globe over await inspiration. An artist
creates a body of work; the cosmetologist might conceive
themselves in this manner by placing ridiculous hairstyles
as objects upon their client's head. Firstly, those styles are
horribly outdated, as the horse-and-buggy were; second,

salon hair is too seldom replicable for women once at home; finally, "hairdos" stay barely perceptible of its natural immaculate state, thrashed by stylists misleading clients, making it practically impossible to repair.

✝

BY JEHR SCHIAVO
WRITING AS GERARD SAINT D'ANGELO

☩

Rock It

Go for it, I'm the generous sort, want to perceive yourself coquettish; bored stiff by one length, mid or long hair; possibly have semi-uncommitted layers; find most days tying yours in a ponytail with some soccer mom baseball cap up top?

Go on now, get some scissors, the pair you cut everything with, don't be a big chicken.

Brush out that snarled ponytail; tip your head down, combing it once again — this time, three-quarters of the way straight forward, just centimeters before resembling a unicorn.

Refasten that elastic band, between the very top of your head and center forehead's hairline.

Everything's even, right, every hair appears combed through snug, leaving that which protrudes from the elastic band?

Okay, spunky one, now bring your head upright.

Hold high by your least dexterous hand the ponytail, in what no time whatsoever can be a keepsake with those feeling sentimental — trash for others completely fed up, pretty much appearing similar to most everybody else.

Point your scissors toward the elastic — no matter what you do, don't make an easy undertaking punishing, accidently cutting that band securing a neat and tidy ponytail, nor fingers or scalp; cuts should be made exclusively to hair.

Avoid chopping straight across the hair; a thatched broom bristle effect isn't what you're after — instead erratically chip, hack, peck into hair's excess length which extends beyond your elastic band.

Remove the elastic band when you believe you're done, cutting itself should take seconds.

What did I tell you — killer, huh? Thick, long wavier hair assumes an Italian B-movie Monica Vitti similarity; shorter, finer texture may resemble Chrissie Hynde, in the gritty style of *Precious*. Any strays, snip them off — better yet, don't bother, imagine them as drips and splatters at the side edges of a fifty-million-dollar Basquiat.

✝

BY JEHR SCHIAVO
WRITING AS GERARD SAINT D'ANGELO

✝

UN FAVORI

Francis Coppola didn't have many choices for the fruit
Marlon Brando stuck between his teeth and lips scaring
that poor little kid — who either acted exquisitely
or reacted perfectly unscripted seconds after Don
Corleone collapsed from sudden cardiac arrest. Virtually
impossible to employ by similar way, the thin skin of
an apple, peach or apricot; lemon peel too bitter —
shooting that scene, take after retake would've been
rough going, even for Brando. Much earlier during this
masterpiece, moments after bumbling Fredo stood by
in horror watching his father plummet against their
car's front hood, grill, and bumper, Marlon finally slid
expertly toward the damp pavement. A few oranges
then rolled out of Corleone's small brown paper sack
which some Asian storekeeper had seconds ago gifted the
Don, who earnestly tried purchasing them at his favored
outdoor fruit stall. A pair of unforgettable *Godfather*
scenes, containing one Marlon Brando and two surprise
elements, using as an essential prop: the orange. Might

the French, possibly Taiwanese, slice orange wedges playing bogeyman for their young family members?— my Uncle Tony did this to me when I was about four, digesting several courses of Jean's homemade Sicilian Sunday afternoon marathon meals.

Here, a place in allusion, partings of merit require that certain red satin bow — exact shade your imagination, with regards to cinching together the goodbye, giving intimacy's sense, as long lost friends reuniting, "However are you, it's been more autumns than I dare confess." Nostalgic Mr. Haute Coiffure, didn't register at the start, when I wrote a metaphor of humans as fruit not falling far from their own that we would revisit this idea again once more. Abstract philosophy by beautician — I must kindle some sort of mutual comprehension, missing an association otherwise could abandon most as Fredo, impressionable yet confused.

What makes me believe mankind and oranges were destined to earth from the single force that, for example, also brought fish, cows, or water — a worthy topic, but dicey; many differ, convinced sea creatures have their separate creative power, as would cattle, along with every other single living thing. I'd prefer permission to agree; everyone disagreeing oranges aren't another blessing from the universe may be excused immediately — a shame, I know, but it's getting late, and arguments quickly eat up any clock.

If I were on a hike galavanting the hillside near Vito Corleone's birthplace, maybe I'd reach up, picking that

orangest Sicilian orange growing from its bountiful tree.
Parched from the arid Mediterranean sun, I'd decide to
squeeze its juice, quenching my thirst, carrying me another
six farm groves back into town. Plan of action: drink
half at a time, divide the orange equally by pocketknife.
Perched upon a respectable boulder in the middle of
Sicily, I couldn't help but notice this moist pulp's color
— brilliance forming from that starburst pattern within
its confines. Heavenly, gone for a quiet holiday, pacing
yourself, leisurely engaged, calculating anything or nothing
whatsoever. In a trice, my palms cupping both halves
treasure this awesome beauty, oranges I've sliced by that
same manner at other locations, each orange also of
unparalleled design, cut evenly on St. Barts, Zingaro, or
Fredo's watery grave, Lake Tahoe.

Would I or willing participants, painting the orange
tree's fruit silver, make them that much more beautiful
than their neighboring virgin citrus tree? Today, from
dawn's beginning in creation's wanderlust, humans, too,
also divine, as such beauty the fish, cow and water. Shall I
brush cerulean blue pigment over a koi fish, careful not to
cover their gills, eyes and mouth? I'll spray a dairy cow's
white hide crimson, placing foils over the black spots,
leaving them unchanged. High above Yosemite's valley
floor, I'd unload drum after drums full of astro-lime-
green-neon dye, producing an antifreeze waterfall.

Potentially, the perpetrator of those crimes would
face hefty penalties, fines, and/or imprisonment. How
it is unethical to prohibit application of toxic poison

desecrating our planet, animals, fish, plants, and water, while performing so-called beauty services using harsh chemicals on perfectly beautiful people remains globally acceptable — questionable conduct by those who possess such power, the licensed cosmetologists. With unusual exception, the hairstylist applying chemicals temporarily loses his or her client; subsequent women, convinced by their obstetrician recently discovering hers was a positive test; she is indeed pregnant, as suspected. This particular patron is advised by her doctor she should hold off until post-delivery before receiving any future chemical service applied in the beauty salon or done at home. Bizarre, she will by large percentages adhere to the obstetrician's suggestion out of trepidation, sheer fright alone protecting her much-adored fetus. However, in great numbers they'll race to make that crucial appointment receiving chemical services almost immediately, days after giving birth, not ever thinking twice those same chemicals warned about nine months earlier could also have harmful effects on mother.

✝

BY JEHR SCHIAVO
WRITING AS GERARD SAINT D'ANGELO

✝

MOBOCRACY

Late June, as every other year, my cosmetologist license must be renewed or expires; whereby, if delinquent after five years an all-day exam — written and practical occurs, following another four-hundred-hour overpriced refresher course in any accredited beauty school, plus additional state fees for their extra effort reissuing a paper license; board approved, I proceed legally.

Before Las Vegas suffered lost revenue during the great 2008 recession I thought having my Nevada cosmetologist license wouldn't be an unwise idea. I paid a certified beauty school in that state affiliated with Nevada's Cosmetology Board, complied with mandatory testing, passed, and received licensing. Taking into account Las Vegas had been beaten up the first three of these last eight years, there was no logical reason to pursue business nor further renewal holding that state's license.

My current license is a valid one, although I've practiced in several states whose board wasn't aware; had they been, none would have recognized the state which does. Since Boards of Cosmetology within the United States refuse to recognize each other, as medicine does, Mr. Haute Coiffure cries protestation's plea unto every licensed cosmetologist living in America. I urge declination of reinstatement upon expiration date; abolish this system, theirs structured on a fuddy-duddy foundation, meeting requirements in standard beauty nearly one hundred years old.

Cosmetology schools, academies and/or beauty colleges ought to shut their doors forever, they absolutely should; those programs are defunct, quite useless. Webster's unblemished definition of cosmetic: "not substantive, insignificant, superficial." This isn't any call for arms. Last I checked, no Board of Cosmetology enlisted private militia; maybe North Korea does, though not many outsiders beyond Dennis Rodman get invitations there to discern verity from fabrication, probably won't myself unless Kim Jong-un requests his Jehrcut — if he does, I'm going, another capitalist providing a communist's extravagant indulgence.

This proposed *coup d'etat* of the beauty machine would cost nothing to a cosmetologist; not paying fees for new applicants or license renewals alongside accrued penalties across these United States will, however, cause an obliterating ripple effect. Don't be distressed, so what, a few state employees at Cosmetology Boards won't find it necessary to punch their time cards any longer, big deal, collateral damage, *c'est la vie*. They should've thought twice before spending lifelong careers examining an applicant's procedure applying ammonium thioglycolate acid, the main ingredient to rearrange hair structure for permanent waves and straighteners, or diaminotoluene, ethanolamine, p-phenylenediamine, potassium persulfate, sodium metasilicate — compounds found in tint, along with bleach.

All poison, I contend, that which slays hair while contaminating the myriad of drains directly flowing into our ecosystem, because these aforementioned widespread chemicals used for beauty services remain legal.

I'm floored at how many people will go out of their way paying top dollar buying organic food, dedicating pantry shelves, overflowing with vitamin supplements, and bathroom areas to cascading "natural, non-toxic, chemical-free" beauty products, but these same individuals have no issue, not ever thinking before yet another harmful, environmentally-unfriendly hair color, bleach, straightener, or permanent wave application.

✝

✝

BOB MARLEY SAID SO

Hippies, among their other innovative topics, objected to a meat-and-potatoes lifestyle alongside similar mentality defiling the environment. Flower power change occurred — took decades, but actually happened, didn't it — recycling trash bins replaced aluminum garbage cans practically everywhere, farmers markets grace neighborhoods offering sustainable organics.

If my opinion holds no weight by reason that Mr. Haute Coiffure lacks scholarly authority, fair enough, I couldn't agree more. "Your honor, may I bring forth before the court my next witness, Dr. Manuela Gago-Dominguez?"

"Doctor, please raise your right hand and solemnly swear or affirm that you will tell the truth, the whole truth and nothing but the truth, so help you God?"

"Alright then, Doctor, is it true your findings which link prolonged permanent hair color usage and cancer were in fact established as a researcher at the University of Southern California?"

"Thank you — now, Doctor, would it also be true hairstylists applying permanent hair color are indeed prone to a higher risk of developing cancer than those clients receiving the chemical service itself?"

"Disquieting if I were a hairstylist, Doctor. Could you then assert clients are without health's jeopardy receiving tints, highlights and lowlights which contain permanent hair color?"

"Stunning, both hairstylists and clients are undoubtedly in danger — what alarming information. Doctor, you've listed breast cancer, gallbladder cancer, bladder cancer and lymphoma, all severe types that possibly connect beauty treatments offered throughout not only this country but the whole civilized world?"

"Your data has been printed throughout scores of medical journals and familiar publications, including one prominent January 29, 2001 *Los Angeles Times* article. These statistics in entirety have been presented before the Food and Drug Administration, National Cancer Institute, alongside our American Cancer Society; each fail to concur with such findings — Doctor, I'm appalled, their neglect is disgraceful, utterly outrageous."

"Your honor, ladies and gentlemen of the jury, there on any cigarette package sold, buyers clearly read that warning labeling smoking's hazard can be fatal; yet some continue to smoke regardless, although fewer than in years past. Wouldn't it be judicious if every salon, beauty supply, and retailer furnishing permanent hair color, post in plain sight an acceptable warning, resembling those signs we typically read within and around common areas of public space that may also cause cancer?"

Hypothetically, after primitive state-run licensing boards and cosmetology institutions of inferior education become vacant, beauty supply stores should be next in line keeling over. Take charge of your income, hairstylists. It's not necessary forking over fifty percent or more of hard-earned wages in commission to salon owners using you, peddling their beauty products at the reception desk. Let's for one minute pretend you're languid, maybe not quite; you've an actual existence other than being under scrutiny forty, fifty, even sixty salon hours each week — work a fraction of those hours, earning parallel salary making house calls.

Scanned the business section recently — real estate, lots of it available, always has and will continue. Suggestions: a maximum four-chair boutique establishment or an exclusive station inside your spare bedroom of that home you lease — even better, the house you're purchasing. Physicians, our highly respected consummate professionals, used to practice in their multiple-storied Victorian front parlors. Clients couldn't care in the least who did the interior design of any five-thousand-square-foot, $1.7 million salon. In fact, most knowledgeable customers frequenting superplex day spa salons understand the majority of their total receipt wasn't solely apportioned toward that establishment's employees serving them.

BY JEHR SCHIAVO
WRITING AS GERARD SAINT D'ANGELO

What should happen to those corporations manufacturing toxic and misleading beauty products, believe it or not, can occur. Hairstylists have a single thread which weaves us together; we can be light years different, but share disposition of unvarnished independence — many choose this occupation as our livelihood for that candid reason alone. Asserting yourself creatively doesn't necessitate being led around by others — state, employer nor purveyor.

✝

✞

Yes Please

Within the first few chapters of that frayed, linen-covered, purged book about hair I've remorse no longer possessing, as also in National Geographic magazines and documentaries, are stories covering indigenous tribes striving for beauty. Through personal encounters I've deduced our culture in certain respects has devolved — specifically, outward personal beauty and its shallow direction. A respectable depth into the bush or rainforest, tribes-people conscientiously etch out elaborate and complex hairstyles employing broken, rusted razor blades, having far superior results in an unaffected way than those I've struggled with attempting countless occasions using spiffy electric clippers. Dyes found from earth, plants, animal secretion as well are mixed, crushed by ancient mortar with pestle, custom blended, altogether chemical-free, impactful tones on Pacific Rim inhabitant, South American or African tribal skin and hair — for my money truly superb imagery. Their primitive sense of self emits an illustrious inner beauty, that which cosmetic corporate giants couldn't replicate even if coerced through extreme torture; neither can clients leaving salons, failing with enormous effort to duplicate what the stylist had done once they return home.

Traveling onto these alongside other unknown faraway locations is often tedious. A rewarding journey can take hours; layovers are inconvenient; godawful, stuck-in-coach, commercial inflight meal service looks and smells atrocious; itty-bitty bathrooms begin to pile up mid-flight, Customs queue after touchdown feels inhumane, like herding sheep; then your baggage wait, wondering if any got lost, jetlagged, daydreaming someone with an authentic smile waits patiently at their climate controlled vehicle outside the nearest arrivals door.

I have a brand-new pair of Japanese shears — bought them several years ago; they've not ever cut a solitary hair's strand. Outrageous, these scissors, might easily be worth what hundreds of natives earn inside a month living in the Amazon, if there's that many remaining when driverless cars soon rule our roadways.

I'm saving that pair for partial retirement on the select coast boasting consistent sarong temperatures. My favorite patrons will come a-calling, some by car, others airplane, staying up to a week if they choose, visiting Jeanette, LouLou and me. Each day we'll convene, eating what's local and fresh during meals outside in the open air. I'll have ample opportunity observing my client's minutest daily hair's cutting; theirs spoken by a southerly breeze yesterday, eastern today, from the north tomorrow, westerly another following day. Shortly around late afternoon's heat subsiding, when the sun soothes behind Matisse clouds, shifting into rosier shades, I'll be holding those shears — for now, safely set aside.

☦

BY JEHR SCHIAVO
WRITING AS GERARD SAINT D'ANGELO

MR. HAUTE COIFFURE

✝

Afterword

Tipping my hat, giving that due nod here would be appropriate pronouncing this in some measure the dedication. If I were most, this could easily be written as something similar to whomever that person is who loves and inspires me, yet would have signified nothing for you after reading *Mr. Haute Coiffure* unless you're family or friend. Outsiders wouldn't have any knowledge, if an inscripted name were Sadie, be her my aunt or cat, nor bother caring much either.

A hushed brewing suddenly burst wide open inside *Newsweek*'s incendiary cover story concerning women's dearth of power in proportionate balance throughout Silicon Valley. Society as a whole takes Sergey Brin and Larry Page seriously, even though various Google concepts appear futuristic while slightly fanciful. Tim Cook has demonstrated enough driving force that Apple presses ahead comfortably, realising they closed 2015 with their earth-shattering $234 billion in revenue. Facebook barely around a dozen years, Mark Zuckerberg also glides forward, confidently understanding our favored social media site has altered entire governments. For all we don't know, he'll soon personally request His Holiness the Dalai Lama and Pope Francis to friend leaders of Al-Qaeda, Boko Haram, Hezbollah, Al-Shabab, Taliban, though it may seem strange, ISIS too — imagine this, world peace brokered by a few Facebook pages.

Google, Apple, Facebook, three global game changers, evidently they've barely scratched the surface; each create jobs exponentially, ten thousand employees a-crack at Google's upcoming 1.9 million square foot Moffett Field campus. Picture Sergey, Larry, Tim or Zuck wearing frumpy haircuts, cuts local newscasters are often seen with, that John Boehner-Ted Cruz button-down hairdo. What if either tech titan's skin tone overnight appeared a bit chalky, simply because their new fake hair tint didn't quite seem right? Suppose twenty-four hours thereafter Sergey, Larry and Tim showed up stupefying all of us with no traces of silver, while Mark excitedly joined in too and began highlighting his hair, disguising any unruly grays. He's currently worth fifty-five billion, but does anyone really take Oracle's Emperor Ellison seriously; between his plastic surgery and Grecian formula hair dye, it's like, wait one second, "What was so wrong your life necessitated that nonsense anyway?"— an aberration, a techie's tragic waste on so many levels.

Sexism, not specifically set aside toward those undulating knolls rolling across Silicon Valley. Should anyone forget those immortal crying lyrics of James

Brown, *this is a man's world, but it wouldn't be nothing without a woman or a girl* — yes, sung nearly five decades ago; although, what about such pertinent discussion among women today, Silicon Valley or elsewhere for that matter? France's Christine Lagarde, Managing Director of the International Monetary Fund, now here's a woman to be reckoned with — striking bones, beautifully tailored subdued suits, makeup barely noticeable, an understated haircut, proudly wearing her natural color, as do Sergey, Larry, Tim, and Mark. Lagarde commands respect; hers is intellect earned, her visual appearance by itself speaks unequivocally, "I'm absolutely confident in who I am."

Nancy Pelosi, on the other hand, should consider hiring a new makeup artist, alongside wardrobe and hair stylists. Her Beverly Hills Hotel luncheon persona might be believable at The Polo Lounge, although honestly she hasn't in my aesthetic judgement resonated credible politics.

I have the same opinion, there's plenty of space for improvement — women do rightly deserve that front plush seat dominating their corporate boardrooms. A forty-year-old woman projecting an unconvincing toe-head blonde she sported during childhood may excel hosting presidential campaign fundraisers in her Peninsula home, but expecting believability that next morning ten minutes away at the boardroom table wearing said tediously maintained, blown-out, bleached bob which momentarily captured admirers' attention during yesterday's glitzy la-dee-da afternoon suddenly loses cachet. Sixty-nine-year-old heavenly songstress Emmylou Harris still belts it out, at ease with having gone totally gray. Like night and day, chanteuse Debbie Harry, pushing seventy, continues bleaching her hair blonde, channeling former glory, Blondie — equivalent to a well-known female Silicon Valley CEO who perpetually bleaches hers.

Women, you're indubitably more than capable — my sisters, you should wield such potential Sergey, Larry, Tim, and Mark hold; how, though, may in point of fact be assisted by taking Lagarde's cue appearing plausible, accompanying your personal distinction along with intellectual capacity.

To whom I dedicate Mr. Haute Coiffure: *those undaunted by the past, constantly proud of their inner beauty, guiding this brief and priceless odyssey, mind, body and spirit.*

✝

Acknowledgement, Credit and Gratitude

Extraordinaire, Eric Doctor, both graphic designer and editor for *Mr. Haute Coiffure*, front through back cover.

Quite supreme bull's eye my first aim — well, actually, second attempt — securing literary and artistic support before publishment. Amazon's automaton publishing partner in reality shouldn't be counted; turned out they didn't require any substantial engagement with me, the author, nor obliged to read this entire manuscript.

Eric Doctor came aboard by a well-founded referral, still I was jittery; he living in Brooklyn, while I'd been on the Pacific Coast of Oaxaca en route to Vietnam. What I figured momentarily could break the ice, was not starting off saying hello by phone, but instead using, "what's up Doc?" Exchanging a few emails prior to our verbal introduction I immediately ruled out the Bugs Bunny jest.

Brilliant would be an understatement; Eric mystifies any cynic's perception this book wasn't shielded by outside angels — he's numero uno.

Eric didn't know it; however, upon initially reading this recognition, I imagine he was surprised to learn I'd thrown an adequate temper tantrum hanging up, following our second meeting over the telephone. Nobody ever made changes for what I'd written; I immaturely took his edits far too harshly.

After some unbridled belligerence I realized yelling American profanity within my Mexican villa would be of no use; alternative choice, pick up the remote, tuning out, turning on television. Sixty-seven channels: a German news editorial program, sixty-two strictly hearing Spanish — I eventually stopped, seeing *The King's Speech* on one of those four remaining stations, fortunately spoken in English.

Let's put it this way: Eric's relationship with me was illuminated minutes into rewatching Geoffrey Rush train Colin Firth. Without Eric Doctor I would stammer; my writing's raw version suffers its unique speech impediment. Ah, luck does at times have its way, King George VI and Lionel Logue remained friends for life. Lots can happen between now and death; Eric (the Doctor) undeniably has had my back; should the situation arise, somehow I'll cover his, *semper fidelis.*

Speaking of covering, what about *Mr. Haute Coiffure*'s graphic identity designed by Eric Doctor — in the immortal words of Rod Stewart and strummer Ronnie Wood, *Every picture tells a story don't it?*

✝

✝

What kind of child gets a crisp salute in her Poppi's book?
One day I'd been the hairstylist-parent, usually around
in our live-work loft; suddenly overnight, within a blink
of an eye, I pretty near vanished — her Poppi's full-time
attention all but gone. LouLou was four-and-a-half in
Miami Beach when Gerard Saint D'Angelo got crackin'
— six manuscripts later on arid Lampedusa, my daughter
was two months away from turning twelve. Not once
throughout these past eight years flitting about globally
has LouLou ever whined, "Poppi, why can't we play now?"
or dramatically complained, "Do you have to work every
day?" However, sure as the day is long, she'd give me a
smooch on one cheek; then upon almost every occasion
add, "good luck." Molding into place my essential Mack's
silicone earplugs; blank white paper beneath pencil
in hand — whipped several hours thereafter I'd hear
LouLou with heartfelt twinkle, probing, "How did it go?"

Imagine your two bestest of friends ever and ever,
theirs are an inconceivable nonstop belief in you.
Truth be known, during my sincerest introspection in
bachelorhood, I never gathered I'd be graced by Jeanette
and LouLou; astounding circumstances can occur — for
me, a kick ass pair of natural-born beauties I'm indulged
to have as family.

✝

✟

Talk about putting yourself on the hot seat. Figures, dopey me, saved the final bit of *Mr. Haute Coiffure* writing 'til now. My impressive wife surely does warrant credit somewhere across this book's cover, but she straight out refused — please join me in a toasty ovation for Jeanette Schiavo. Her considerate prowess was offered at every turn during this particular project, bringing into fruition my collection of essays: from initial #2 lead's drafting entanglement onto digital format; a meticulous husband's umpteen rewrites; our dozen or so pre-edits done in tandem — superwoman Jeanette, presently orchestrating those additional individuals who will propel this project, while always, without fail, reminding me why.

Deep down, the most significant reason I dreamed Jeanette would possibly accept me as a lifetime partner — she thoroughly believes with undying confidence our days together are those hours feeling ideal for her too.

I don't gaze toward the sky without thinking of her any longer; I'll inspect any horizon wondering when Jeanette's favorite cloud might soon drift by. More than likely not so much brains, leaving sole fortuity — one of life's greatest treasures was remaining single until August 22, 2002 — not our wedding date, but Jeanette's first knock at my garden salon door. I'd been struck by her, both thunder and lightning; hers was a defining presence as none other before. From that split second forward I earnestly hoped to be her Rock of Gibraltar — by such finesse Dr. North Shore delivered to his precious wife, Jeanette for eternity shall remain my Mrs. North Shore.

✟

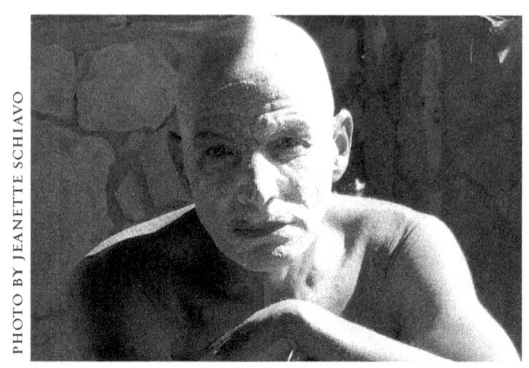

PHOTO BY JEANETTE SCHIAVO

JEHR SCHIAVO is a celebrated hairstylist and raconteur who for nearly four decades has challenged the conventional wisdom of the beauty industry. He and his work have been recognized in *Allure*, *Details*, *Elle*, *The New York Times*, and *Vogue Italia*. He presently travels the world with his wife Jeanette and daughter LouLou, and delivers chic, effortless, healthy, sustainable Jehrcuts to select patrons who commission him in Los Angeles, New York, and San Francisco.

WWW.JEHRSCHIAVO.COM